Changing the Generations

My Journey to Holistic Living

By: Laura B. Hill

Revised, Jan 2024

We wouldn't be the persons that we are without the journeys we go on. Thank you to my husband, Craig Hill, the absolute love of my life. You've supported me through the good and bad. Thank you to my children; Mike and Jess, Joe and Susie, Tara, and Dan. You inspire me more than you will ever know. Thank you to our mothers and fathers, who gave their best.

Above everything else, all praise is to God, the Almighty.

"Plant good seeds and good things shall grow."

Forward
by Craig T. Hill

Sometimes in life you meet someone you never want to walk away from. Laura was just that. An independent thinker, a caregiver to strangers, and a leader with her family.

Laura studied many religions looking for answers to life's questions. She believed the answer to many religious question is found within ourselves. Love for her family has always been her strength .

Her strength was tested when her only daughter received a cancer diagnosis. She focused every waking minute learning and praying and teaching others about nutrition and environment. How we can stop disease before it's too late. Working closely with doctors of all practices she was able to give Tara three more years of a wonderful life. The loss of Tara brought even more life to my wife, Laura, and

her passion to teach others about nutrition and
health.

Table of Contents

Disclaimer

I am not a doctor, a chemist, nor a dermatologist. I am a certified Holistic Nutritionist and Health Coach, sharing my opinion of life experiences and what I was taught in the AFPA certification program, who wants to provide a more natural and healthy lifestyle for my family and others. The information contained on the Honey Hill Naturals, Inc., or blog websites, including but not limited to all workout plans, nutritional advice, and healthy lifestyle tips, is provided for informational purposes only, and is not meant to substitute for the advice provided by your doctor or other qualified health care practitioner. The information available on or through the Honey Hill Naturals newsletters, or (including, but not limited to, information that may be provided by writers, editors, healthcare and/or nutrition professionals employed by, or contracting with, Honey Hill Naturals, Inc., and / or their associates), is not intended to diagnose or treat any disease or prescribe medication. Information and statements regarding dietary supplements or ailments on any of the above sites or newsletters, may not have been evaluated by the Food and Drug Administration (FDA) in the United States of America.

Introduction

I hear cheers and a lot of hootin' and hollerin' coming from the other room. It's Sunday afternoon and our favorite football team is playing on the TV set. The whole family is over, some neighbors too. I'm in the kitchen cooking up some grub. I've got some nachos with the works; ground beef, melted cheese, sour cream, hot peppers, and guacamole. In the deep fryer, I've got a handful of breaded mozzarella cheese sticks bubbling away. Mini sausages in barbeque sauce, deviled eggs, and let's not forget about all the beer in the fridge. We had enough whiskey shots going around that could put any Irish wedding to shame!

What can I say? It was sad, really. This was a very typical weekend for us. I was just happy when I was drinkin'. I didn't see how badly my decisions were affecting my health. I come from a huge Irish family. There are twelve of us. I'm number nine in the rank. Almost all of us were drinkers and smokers. I was downing the beers as early as my pre-teens. (Sssshhhh…my parents don't know that.) This, paired with the unhealthy eating, did not make for a good mix. By the time I was in my mid-thirties, though I could hang with the big boys at the bar, I was severely overweight, pre-hypertensive, and probably pre-diabetic. I was not on a healthy path, and I was most definitely feeling it! My family was suffering from this too. It was most definitely time for a change. When our youngest son suffered a grand mal seizure at twelve years old with no previous condition of it, we had no idea just how much of a change was coming. He was diagnosed with cortical dysplasia with epilepsy. I finally came to terms with this. I knew it was time for me to get myself well and change the generations of my family. I no longer wanted to be the "Irish family that eats and drinks too much".

I cleaned up my act. My husband and I lost weight, quit drinking and smoking and we started working out. We lost almost 50 pounds each! Then, one year later, another big change happened. Our daughter was diagnosed with Ewing's Sarcoma of the chest wall. I'm sorry but there is nothing that prepares you for that wake-up call.

My daughter's cancer journey took us on a three-and-a-half-year course that taught us many lessons, to which I couldn't be more grateful. I suffered through depression, grieving, chronic fatigue syndrome, menopause, auto-immune response causing gluten sensitivity, insulin resistance, weight gain, frozen shoulder, back, hip, and knee pains, pinched nerve in my neck and Achilles tendonitis in both ankles. It was time for another re-boot, and this was where I learned the greatest amount of knowledge. In order to change the generations of my family and make a big enough impact that would stick, I needed to become an expert at it. But where to start?

I found out just how much sugar impacts our health and bodies, especially in conditions like epilepsy, cancer, and even menopause. We were still eating too much of it!

I'm not recommending that you follow any of the guidelines I have mentioned in these pages. We all have our journeys to take. I only share my journey in hopes that it can help you or someone you know, who's wanting to change, and thus change the generations of their family.

Did you know that children's cancer rates are the highest they've ever been? There was a time when getting cancer was an old-person's disease. Not a young-person's disease. Have you ever thought about why that is? I have. I don't believe that it's all genetic. Our government put out an article on PubMed (NIH) stating that only about 5% - 10% of all cancers are actually hereditary. The other 90% - 95% are due to lifestyle choices. I wince when someone tells me they have hypertension or diabetes type 2 because it's hereditary. The CDC states, "6 in 10 Americans have a chronic disease. 4 in 10 have more than one."

Chronic diseases like diabetes and prediabetes, arthritis, heart disease, Alzheimer's disease, cancer, and stroke are common preventable diseases, according to the CDC. Even more interesting is that they tell us the key lifestyle risks for these chronic diseases come from poor nutrition and lack of physical activity!

I believe it has much to do with the toxic, stressful world we created to live in and it's not entirely our fault. Our food and products have been hijacked. However, there is still hope. When we take responsibility for our own health, we become accountable, and we understand what we are up against. Then, we can become better.

We can take better care of the environment we live in. We can stop using so many plastic straws, plastic water bottles, plastics in general as well as paper products that not only pollute our bodies, but also pollute and destroy the earth. We can stop being so connected to our cell phones and Wi-Fi; stop being so dependent on the internet and the use of so many electronics that's causing high EMF's in the air. Stop spraying Round-up and weed killers; we can get out there and pull our own weeds as much as we can. (The very least, it's terrific exercise!) We can eat naturally and organically grown foods instead of food-like items bought in plastic and boxed containers. It's all about the nutrition. This is what our body understands. My mother always said to eat a variety. I believe this is a great way to think. Otherwise, why would God have created so many different foods in such a vast variety for us to eat? I say enjoy it! (Just be mindful of how much you're eating.)

I became a certified holistic nutritionist and health coach with a plethora of information on natural therapies, healthy living, and informed conventional care to help deliver the message that is my daughter's, Tara Hill's, legacy; to help others and myself to live more naturally, age better, and to just be healthier. I became a self-proclaimed expert at all things holistic! Sometimes, I may direct the attention toward benefits for a family. Other times, I may direct it toward menopausal women, or older men and women in general. The holistic information I am sharing relates to all people, in my humble opinion. You can use it all or pick and choose what you wish.

I didn't always pay attention to my health the way I should have. All of that has now changed. Being healthy isn't just about being a size two, ladies. Let the weight loss be a side effect of your good, healthy living. One step at a time; one day at a time. This is where you start. With yourself.

I am always asked about what things I changed in my life in order to live a healthier lifestyle. I can't wait to share it with you! Now, you can read on to find out more of what I did to get back to health, that can now be passed on

to your children, generation after generation!

Chapter One:

The Holistic Life Pyramid

Many people run and hide when they hear the word "holistic". They're not quite sure what that really means, although they know there's the word "organic" tossed around in there. Sounds expensive is another expression I hear all too often. What's expensive are those drive up windows of fast burgers, fast tacos, and fast fries. It may be cheap at the register but trust me on this, your body will pay the price in medical bills later.

My introduction to holistic living was more of a shove, really. I guess I'm the type that needs to be pushed because, Lord knows, I seem to take the long way around in a heartbeat! I was raised with healthy eating on the forefront; that is my mother always had a pretty decent green thumb growing up and her gardens were nothing short of amazing. I always said I didn't inherit her green thumb. We didn't eat out that much back in those days; it was far too expensive. Our snacks seemed to be different as well. My mother made most of our treats and breads from scratch. We didn't even have cell phones or the electronics that we do now, so emf risk was much lower. So, being healthy overall seemed to be a simpler task than today's parents have to deal with. I'm always striving to be as good a mother as I had; I am the mother of four children, though they are grown now. I have three boys (who have some pretty amazing significant others) and one girl, not in that order. A wise man once told me, "If you plant good seeds, then only good things shall grow." If my family is my garden, then my mother's green thumb I indeed inherited!

What I have learned through my journey to holistic living is that the only real cure to any disease is to not get it in the first place. That's a harsh reality for all of us who are steady on the "American diet". When I was younger, I was always active. I played on many team sports at school. I didn't think fast food burgers and fries would make that much of a difference in my life. Until I was thirty-something. Then, my forties came. I found myself eating like that Sunday afternoon all the time, and I didn't like my body. I didn't like how I was feeling. I was sweating all the time and always out of breath.

Truth be told, about half of Americans today believe that it's far easier to complete their taxes each year than it is to eat healthy. That's crazy to think! What is the American diet anyway? Well, it's foods that are highly processed, with a high sugar load, empty calories, and lots and lots of chemicals. Sounds delish, right? Most everything processed contains chemicals and/or sugars that keep us addicted and coming back for more. This way of eating is not only bad for ourselves, but also for the environment as well, with all the garbage and waste they create!

I would like to clarify that any time I refer to holistic "diet' or "diet" in general, I am referring to the simple meaning that diet is all the foods a person eats on a continual or every day basis. I don't want this being equal to "being on a diet" because that is not my intention.

What does living a holistic life mean and why do I say pyramid? Living a holistic life means to live your life in such a way that is as natural to you as well as to your environment in which you live. It is all parts of the self - balanced and connected; mind, body, and spirit. In other words, along with eating healthy, a holistic life also includes what we're thinking and what we're doing. Nutrition alone is just not enough to keep us healthy. We must include the needs of the mind, our energy, our emotions, and spirit along with the body. With that being said, it's about eating organic, whole foods while omitting as much of the junk and processed foods out. Holistic living is very much all about the quality of life. Holistic nutrition is all about the much deeper, interconnectedness of all these parts, that make up the whole. It is a full-body approach indeed!

I say pyramid not because I'm trying to reinvent the wheel here, but because of the concept it represents. The analogy I loved that one of my best friends used for her own business years ago went something like this. Think of the way a pyramid is stacked. You have your bottom or base layer. Then, your next layer staggered on top in a shorter fashion, and the third layer staggered on top of that one in a shorter fashion and so on. If you look at each layer, even though the uppermost layers are shorter in length and maybe not so prominent or important, they're all very important in making the whole. Without all pieces holding firm in all of the layers, the entire pyramid would have holes and be unbalanced. A holistic, healthy life is one that nourishes and takes care of every layer, or the whole human body. We need to try to aim for balance as much as we possibly can. I guess you can imagine an eternity symbol or a circle to represent the same idea.

When my husband, Craig, was in his twenties, he was diagnosed with high blood pressure. He reluctantly took his medicine and just shrugged it off, saying hypertension runs in his family and he was just destined to suffer from it. Decades later, as we discovered the truth, that hypertension is not a hereditary condition and is very much food and lifestyle related, he made a few changes. He changed the foods that he was eating to healthier ones, stopped smoking, and drinking alcohol, and began exercising. As the pounds came off, so did his need for the medication. Within three months, he was completely off the hypertensive meds. To this day, he remains living with healthy blood pressure.

When my daughter was diagnosed with cancer, she was adamant about eating clean and doing natural therapies. This is the pivotal point in my journey where I learned so much knowledge about what it truly means to eat clean and live holistically. It's not just about eating organic whole foods and omitting the pesticide sprayed foods. Though, this is the perfect place to start. Many people tell me they just don't want to give up what they're eating. They don't care, they say, because it tastes good. I always say we choose our own poison.

Have you ever said to yourself? "I have the immune system of a sloth. I get sick easily and often, and it sticks around for a long time. It seems I can never get rid of it." Choosing to take the following steps listed in this book will strengthen your immune system! I rarely become sick with colds and flus, and if I do, they run through my system quickly and easily.

It all starts with the willingness and want to change. These changes I made were accomplished over several years' time, so go at your own pace. If you're basically healthy and want to make changes, you don't need to change overnight. However, if you or a loved one was given a diagnosis of say cancer, then I recommend changing overnight. Receiving a strong diagnosis like cancer is most definitely a wake-up call telling you that you need to make changes urgently.

Chapter Two:
Self-Love/Active Self-Care

Let's start with something seemingly simple; love the skin you're in. Do you feel a little corny when someone talks about self-love? Even a little shy maybe? Awkward? Self-love is the first step of achieving true, active self-care. We first must understand how to really love ourselves. I chose self-love and self-care to be the base, or most important level, of all because of the importance I feel that it is. It is the root of all happiness. It affects our thoughts, our body chemistry, hormones and processes, our energy, and even how we respond to every day stimulus. We are more likely to care about the food we are eating, from a nutrition stand-point, when we are in a state of self-love.

Self-care is the act of performing certain behaviors that allows us to improve our physical and mental well-being. It is one of my most favorite things I do in taking care of myself. Productive self-care will help us provide a balance between the over-stimulation of this ever-busy world and good health. Personally, I don't think we do enough of it.

We may have odd feelings when it comes to self-love because we've always been taught that so much of what's on the outside, is what's important. So, if you're not skinny enough, or pretty enough, or popular enough, or smart enough, and so on…you get the picture; then we're not good enough to love.

Our feelings are even more slighted because we're taught that if we don't love these types of traits in other people as we would like them in ourselves, then we are just being jealous or caddy. Or, my favorite, self-care is often considered to be selfish, shallow, or conceitful. The cycle is never ending.

Filling up our own cup so-to-speak, is priority in self-care. How do you do this? Don't give a hoot what anyone else thinks of you! It is none of your business! I've been told I'm not tall enough to do what I want to do. I've been told I'm not thin enough to do what I want to do. Though these people may have meant well, it's their own perceptions of the weaknesses they have within themselves that are manifesting. I choose not to believe them. This is a resistance of their own, and as we know true of this universe, that which we resist, will persist.

Since the universe is not going to give me a different body, I choose to love how short I am. I love my weight issues. I love my health issues that I have encountered because it gives me the experience and knowledge to help others. I understand and can better feel what someone may be experiencing themselves. Loving yourself is just so important!

The power of self-love will empower you, giving you complete confidence, lifting you to a higher vibrational energy. The healing power of self-care will motivate you, giving you better focus on goals. It's about self-development and personal growth. I spoke about how I used the power of self-care through the grieving process in my first book, *Tara's Choice; A Mother-Daughter Cancer Journey.* I used self-care practices to lift me from the depression that comes from losing a child.

Productive self-care can really come to the rescue. What are some things you can do for self-care? Do you have any favorite things that you do each day or each week? We can do things like reading a good book, journaling, and meditating. We can breathe in some good essential oils or aromatherapy. I just love essential oils and all kinds of oils really. Spoil yourself with a luxurious bath or steamy shower. Turn up the music and dance around the room. We can do something as simple as getting outside, take a walk or just sit and enjoy nature. I have a friend who just loves to walk through her forest preserve area, find a quiet bench somewhere, and read the day away. It doesn't matter to her if it's a good book or interesting magazine. On summer days, I love just getting out and swing for a while on my hammock. It whisks away all the stress of the day. Finding something funny or watching a funny movie is great self-care. This may help to diminish stress also. Laughter is the best medicine, is it not?

Some other productive self-care behavior is doing things like giving to a charity, volunteering, or paying it forward. De-clutter your closet/room/house. Work on relationships; fixing what may be broken or getting rid of them all together. This is about learning when to take a break, when to say yes, or no, and when and where to set up boundaries. Be mindful and know what you need. If you don't do this for yourself, you can bet yourself that no one else is going to!

My favorite things I like to do is a good workout, especially first thing in the morning. If I'm not feeling up to working out, then I do some stretching, qigong, or meditate. I like to keep up with my prayers, read the Qur'an, and other spiritual acts. I like to get myself all cleaned up and showered, ready for the day. I tidy up my room and make my bed. (Yes, make your bed.) I enjoy crafting, whether it's making my natural products, sewing some new clothes, or just scrapbooking. I enjoy all kinds of crafting, which is also a great de-stressor! We are only given one body; let's take care of it.

Did you know that lack of self-care can be one of the reasons we don't lose weight, or even the cause of gaining weight? Self-care includes things like de-stressing, re-focusing, calming anxiety to improve sleep, exercising, eating well, and boosting mental power. When all of these falls out of balance, our body not only holds on to those extra pounds, but also increases our BMI. These trigger hormones like ghrelin and leptin in a negative way. Ghrelin is a hunger-stimulating hormone. When out of balance, ghrelin says, "Hey! We're hungry!" Leptin is a hormone that tells our brain we're not hungry; that we've had enough to eat and we're full. When Leptin is out of balance, it says, "Wait a minute! Did we eat anything today? We better keep eating to be sure." Cortisol is a hormone that gives us energy. When we have a constant flow of cortisol, we develop insulin-resistance which stops us from burning fat, especially in our belly.

Taking care of my health is another huge part of my self-love, self-care regimen. Eating good foods are full of good energy, and that energy transfers to you. You will read more about that in the next chapter. I like to keep up with chiropractic treatments and adjustments. Chiropractic medicine believes that all body processes are supplied by the nerves that run through the spine, and if there are blockages where those nerves cannot deliver the messages properly, that's when ailments begin. I believe this too. I feel so much better when my neck and back are in good alignment. I also enjoy doing far-infrared saunas to detox and release stress, along with drinking green juices. All that good energy makes me feel so good.

The point being, there are just numerous things we can do. When all is said and done, self-love and self-care really means putting yourself first. It means to get real with yourself, with what you like to do or not to do. It's a knowing of what gives you great energy and what takes it away.

If you saw yourself sitting by yourself in a room full of people, and everyone was just buzzing around doing what they do. Let's say you saw yourself dirty, hair messed up, clothes just dingy and hanging on you. And you could tell you were hungry and thirsty. Would you want to take care of this person? What would you offer? Would you want to clean him/her up? How would you dress this person? Would you want to feed him/her? What would you feed this person? I'm guessing you would show love and concern to this person. So why would taking care of yourself need any less loving action?

Mindfulness creates discipline. I'll probably say this a hundred more times in this book because I think it is that important! It doesn't matter how many times you go to the gym or how great of a workout you do, you can still be overweight and diseased if you're not watching what it is that you're doing the rest of the day. Does this make sense? Be mindful of how you take care of yourself, in all of your habits. The discipline will come when you start to see that if you truly loved yourself, you wouldn't eat badly, dress badly, speak badly, or think badly.

Let's be honest. I think there is something in self-care that makes a woman truly, so beautiful. Be that woman! If you're a man, the same goes for you. Self-care makes a man irresistible and drives women crazy. Be that man!

Chapter Three:

The Holistic Diet

Let's do a quick discussion about how our bodies work, shall we? You will enjoy this, trust me. First, what I have found in people as we try to embark on a healthy eating plan is not lack of will-power. Oh no. People are actually very strong-willed. We first think that if we fail on a diet, that we don't have any will-power. I think this is just nonsense. We all are equipped with an amazingly strong will-power! What I find lacking is that we have our brains set on default mode.

Scientists discovered in the 1990's, a default mode network, or DMN for short, within our brains. This DMN is active when we aren't doing much of anything; that is when our activities don't demand too much of our attention. So, how does this affect our daily eating plan? It's my opinion that we only lack mindfulness. Mindfulness is simple. It's achieving a mental state of one's awareness, focused on the present moment. That means to be present and conscious with how your feeling, especially when food or meal times are concerned. Every so often, throughout your day, check in with yourself. Notice your surroundings. How are you feeling? What are you thinking about? Be present in the moment and observe your "self". We can do that, right?

How many of us make a quick bite to eat for dinner that's made from something boxed or frozen? How many of us don't even take the time to cook a homemade meal, and purchase something from a fast food restaurant? Even if all we have to cook for is our own selves, why do we not bother? Yet, if we were cooking a meal for our mother or father, or one child, we would make them a nice big spread to eat?

Then, we park ourselves in front of the TV to watch some mindless show? I'm not talking about emergencies or extraordinary circumstances here. Just every day routines. When we eat like this, we are eating in the default mode. We're not being mindful of our food, or how many bites we're taking, or if we're even chewing our meal. We only need to be aware of how we are eating to get our brains out of default mode. Observe that you have not been mindful, and that you've been living on default mode. Becoming your own witness to this will began to make a shift, that will make you better at mindfulness. It will become a habit, like second nature.

Second, I learned something very interesting about how our stomachs work. Our bodies are amazing, and they know what we need. In very laymen's terms, it goes like this. You see, our stomachs have what is called a stretch factor, as well as having nutrient receptors. Have you ever eaten something really healthy like some raw celery and carrot sticks with some green juice and felt satisfied until your next meal, and another time you have a fast food burger, fries and a shake and feel like you can still eat more? This would happen to me, often.

When we eat healthy, wholesome, raw, and real foods, our stomach works like a computer, scanning each ingredient and nutrient, or calorie. As the bag (our stomach) fills up, it stretches. The stretch factor lets our brains know that we are full. Then our stomachs are able to perform what it needs to in order to disperse and metabolize our meal. When we eat a highly processed meal full of sugars and bad fats (i.e., the American diet), our stomachs fill up but is not able to "read" most of the products we just gave it. So, the stretch factor is thrown off and cannot figure out when to tell our brains that we are full…so we keep eating because we don't feel satisfied.

Now that we understand these two things, it's plain to see that we can easily manage a healthy eating plan. Don't you think?

Let me throw something out at you. We need to stop with the fad diets and start living right! We must hold ourselves accountable. Yo-yo diets and fads, with their quick weight-loss promises and suddenly six pack abs in two weeks, is just not going to fit the bill. We, especially for us women, though some men experience this also, as we reach our older and wiser selves, continue with this body-shaming cycle. We look in the mirror and find that our clothes don't seem to fit the same way they used to. We notice our muscle tone has gone down despite doing the same workouts we have always done. We expect to be a size 4, or for men, may expect to keep the same muscle-bound physique. I see so many people who try these diets for many reasons.

Bottom line is, they don't have lasting success and they're not healthy for our systems.

We require different amounts of nutrients, especially as we get older, like calcium, vitamin D, Potassium, and vitamin B12 for example. The makeup of our body is ever changing, so it makes sense that we will need different amounts of nutrients to support homeostasis. I'm here to encourage you to eat for your health (and age), then your size and physique will naturally fall into a healthy, good-looking, attractive state. I know that we are barraged by cheap processed foods on the daily, but I know we can do better. It only takes a little bit of commitment to yourself to get the ball rolling in the right direction. So, let's stop with the fad diets. We must be responsible and take more care about what/how/when we are eating. Then, you will find, you're not going to have it any other way.

What is your idea of a holistic eating plan? I think it should consist of foods that are minimally processed, unrefined, or as close to the natural state as possible. It's my opinion that it should be foods that are organic and non-gmo as much as possible. Locally grown foods, as well as fruits and veggies grown in your own garden work well also. These types of foods support our well-being, giving us optimal nutrition and support for growth and repair of tissues.

Want to know about how to shop organically? What I always suggest, is to take things in increments. What we did when we were switching over to organic eating was to learn about labels and how to read them. We learned to follow the dirty and clean dozen list by EWG. Learning the labels mean to know what organic means versus natural, and, also about non-gmo's, high fructose corn syrup and other chemicals and substances that shouldn't be in our foods. You'll become a pro at it; trust me. Sometimes we can't get a product in organic, but they have the non-gmo or the conventional product. I would then choose to get the non-gmo product.

The dirty and clean dozen is a list of produce put out by EWG, or Environmental

Working Group. The dirty dozen list tells us the produce that has the highest amount of pesticides on them, and they put out this list every year. I always look forward to it. Produce on the dirty list, these we buy organic for sure. The clean list is the list of produce that tells us it's ok to buy conventionally. If there was a produce item on the clean list that we ate all the time, however, then I would buy that organic instead. So, for example, broccoli is not on the dirty dozen list so that makes it okay to buy conventional, but we eat it several times a week. I would buy this organic because I didn't want to take chances with the pesticides. When buying conventionally grown produce, remember to wash them well to get off as much of the pesticide residue as possible.

Are you aware that our foods also carry a vibrational energy? High vibrational foods are extremely nutritious for us. These are foods made by God, not processed foods or food from fast food restaurants. We say *If God made it, you're good to go. If man made it,* RUN! Let's get down to the foods then, shall we?

These foods are of course, generally good for anyone as we are all requiring the nutrients from these foods. There are, after all, one hundred percent of humans eating foods of some sort to stay alive. We might as well be eating the best foods for our well-being!

My mother raised me with the belief that eating a variety is best. I live by this theory today because our bodies get used to routine so quickly. Eating a variety ensures that we are getting the most nutrients that are offered from the different foods. Here's what my family and I eat for optimal health and what I generally recommend as a health coach:

It is recommended by functional docs to eat at least six to nine cups of **organic or locally grown vegetables and some fruits** per day. This can easily be done by eating a nice big salad (about four cups of greens) or two smaller salads (about two cups of greens) every day. I make only one rule to this for myself: you must eat the salad before you eat your meal. This gets that proper stomach stretch and the right hormone (Leptin) triggered. Then, add other toppings like other veggies, beans, peppers, mushrooms, tomatoes, cheeses, eggs, dried fruits; even your favorite salad dressing! Sprinkle your salad with a little vinegar or use vinegar-based salad dressings as vinegar improves insulin sensitivity. You can do this, right? I want you to *enjoy* these salads. If you need to train your taste buds to eat sour foods like vinegar, then you can do that, too. I say enjoy your favorite salad dressing, for example, while you're building up this practice of healthier eating. The good, in my opinion, outweighs the bad. Also, habits will stick better when you can go at your own pace to practice them.

Eat vegetables with every meal. Eat whole fruits; not canned and limit fruits to two to three servings per day, because of their usually high sugar content (most berries excluded). Whole fruits are naturally balanced with fiber and natural sugars, called fructose. This balance allows a steadier flow of sugars in the body to prevent insulin spikes.

Now, with that being said, fructose may not be the right thing for you. There are some people who can handle eating more fruit; I'm just not one of them. I feel that because I have such a sweet tooth, I tend to leave out many of the needed veggies because I'm always looking for something sweet instead.

Dr. Lustig explains we consume far too much fructose on a daily basis. Dr. Robert H. Lustig, M.D., M.S.L. is Professor emeritus of Pediatrics, Division of Endocrinology at the University of California, San Francisco (UCSF). He suggests we should only consume 25 grams of fructose daily.

Something else you I must share with you is about eating greens. Greens have an immense impact on our bodies, our gut, and health. I always say it's about the nutrition, but greens go beyond nutrition. You must know that greens have the power to boost our immune system, enhance our gut biome and decrease bloating. Greens increase cognitive function (yes, veggies make you smarter) and are crucial in the detoxification process of our liver. Are you one that depends on coffee, sugary treats, or endless Monster drinks to keep you going? Greens gives our bodies a natural energy production. Eating your veggies also aid in losing and/or maintaining a healthy weight. Greens literally affect every system in our bodies on a cellular level!

Again, I *always* suggest eating your salad and veggies *before* you eat the rest of your meal. This will get that stretch factor going in your stomach and preparing to tell your mind that you're full. Fresh organic foods naturally taste better and have more value where nutrients are concerned, than ones sprayed with pesticides and herbicides. Genetically modified (gmo) foods are not safe for us to consume because of the many health problems they cause, as well as damage to animals and the environment.

If you don't like vegetables or find it just too hard to get that many servings in, making green smoothies (blending) or juicing greens may be the answer for you. These methods make the veggies much tastier and easier to get down. I first started juicing when my daughter had cancer. She would have four 8-12-ounce juices a day! I would have one to two a day. My favorite way lately has been to make green smoothies. Whichever way you choose, you can't go wrong. You can get as much as fifteen servings in just one quart of juiced or blended greens! This will more than satisfy your veggie quota for the day. Another way I look at it is, is that by using these methods, besides getting in huge amounts that would be hard to eat, you also get in greens like Swiss chard, beet tops, and kale, that you wouldn't normally eat on a regular basis. Start off with smaller batches and work your way up to about a quart a day. I'm absolutely amazed with the changes in my own body and health because of doing this! And my skin looks so radiant!

If you're not able to do all those veggies, you might want to look into the proper way of eating carnivore. This way of eating also holds many benefits for good health as well.

If you eat meat, only eat **organic, grass-fed meats and pasture-raised dairy** that do not contain hormones or antibiotics. Remember, if the animal is getting hormones and antibiotics, you will be getting those hormones and antibiotics as well. Sounds delish, right? Not! Women especially have lots of hormonal issues to tend with. We don't need to add any more to the mix. I really felt this fact more around that blessed time of the month, and even more so when I was going through menopause.

Animal products do have some really great health benefits as well, not just drawbacks. My daughter and I had our blood profiles checked when we were eating vegan. We found that our systems were not able to get the required vitamin B12 and iron levels from plants. Years later, I found out that I carry the MTHFR gene. This is a gene mutation that is centered around methylation and requires vitamin B12, folate (not folic acid), and magnesium, as well as other B vitamins, choline, zinc, and so on. It may be a good idea for you to have your own blood profile checked if you're not feeling well on an all plant-based or animal-based diet.

To know how much protein your body needs, I use the following formula. Take your current weight and multiply this by 0.36. This number becomes your minimum amount of protein grams *per day*. Then, take your current weight and multiply by 0.7. This number is the minimum amount of protein grams you need *per day*. Example: 180 x 0.36 = 64.8. 180 x 0.7 = 126. So, this person can eat between 65 and 126 grams of protein per day, spread out in each meal. (It's best to spread protein out in each meal and not all at once because protein can turn to sugar in the body.)

What is currently being recommended by doctors in this space is actually much simpler than what's stated above. Very simply, you can calculate your protein by using the formula of *one gram of protein per every pound of ideal body weight*. So, this would go as follows; if you are a person who currently weighs 200 pounds and you want to weigh 150 pounds, you would eat 150 grams of protein throughout the day. If your goal weight changes to 135 then, you would be reaching for 135 grams of protein per day. So much easier, am I right?

When eating pastas, rice, breads, and cereals, choose **whole grains**. Keep portions under control. Eating too many carbs will most likely result in weight gain. I also try to swap out for sprouted whole grains whenever possible. If any of these products have the word *enriched* in the ingredients, it's a good indication that the product was highly processed and is void of most of the nutrients it started out with. This is especially important if you also have the MTHFR gene. It is said that all grains in America have been sprayed with folic acid, which those of us with this gene mutation, have a tougher time methylating this synthetic nutrient. Aim for grains that state they have not been enriched.

I try to eat carbohydrate foods earlier in the day because even if they don't contain sugars outright, our bodies turn them into sugar. I remember as a young girl, being very active and athletic, my coach would always give that big speech. Do you know which one I'm talking about? It's the "go home and have your mom make you a super big plate of spaghetti for dinner so you have lots of energy for tomorrow's track meet." Or "Fill up on breads and carbs so you have energy for tomorrow's gymnastic meet." Yeah…no. I don't recall being fueled up. I remember being bloated and tired. Gone are the days of eating heavy carb meals for dinner. Eat those early so you're sure to burn off the sugar before it gets stored as fat. (In the case of insulin resistance or MTHFR, I try to restrict carbs as much as possible.)

Another aspect of the 15/6 rule that you'll read about a little further on is used here also. (As in the Belly Fat Cure.) Have you heard of this rule before? If you're a woman, I'm almost certain you have. I think it's a great tool to use. Here's how it works for carbs and sugars.

Keep the sugar grams you eat at 15 grams or less per day. (1 gram of sugar = 1 serving.) Use the following carb chart to keep track of the carbohydrate servings per meal. Stay at 6 or less servings per day. So, for example, if your meal contains 40 grams of carbs, that would equal 2 servings for the day so far.

Get yourself a handy journal if you need to, to keep track. I love journaling for so many reasons, but especially for tracking food intake and such. Our chances for success is greatly improved when we're writing down progress and goals. I created my own journals that do just that!

Carbohydrate Conversion Chart

Grams-Low	Grams-High	Servings
0	4	0
5	20	1
21	40	2
41	60	3
61	80	4
81	100	5
101	120	6

Healthy fats! We need healthy fats in our diet. These contain essential fatty acids that our bodies need to absorb nutrients like fat-soluble vitamins A, D, E, and K, as well as antioxidants. We need Omega-3 fats to support cell structures for function of nerves, brain, and heart. The standard American diet is too high in Omega-6 fats. Ideally, we need a balance of Omega-3 to Omega-6. When taking out junk foods, processed carbs and refined sugars from your diet, the addition of healthy fats is recommended. Healthy fats like nuts and seeds, avocado, grass-fed butter or ghee, nut butters, whole fat creams and dairy, fatty fish, and eggs, as well as healthy oils like coconut, olive, avocado oil, and even dark chocolate will help to keep you feeling more satisfied.

The role of healthy fats is to help maintain a steady metabolism which boosts us into fat-burning mode. They help to support hormones in the body, support cell growth, help to protect our organs and they help our body to absorb nutrients. They're also filling.

What does this mean? It means that adding fats to your meals will keep you fuller longer, so you can make it to your next meal without having to snack in between. Which, of course, means we lower insulin-resistance, thus burning fat as fuel instead of sugar. Fats also gives us younger-looking skin and healthy hair and nails. Now who doesn't want that?

The best way to add these fats into your diet is by adding them into your meals or smoothies. A good rule of thumb to figure how much of these fats you should eat goes like this; if you want to weigh 180 pounds, you could eat as much as 90 grams of fat. (Take 180 x 0.5 grams = 90 grams.) So, it would be 30 grams, or about 2 tablespoons, per meal. You would keep adjusting this number as you keep adjusting your goal weight.

Life is about joy and variety. I believe our food should be too if that's what you like. I recommend eating a **variety** of raw and minimally processed foods that you like because that's how my mom raised me. We have better health overall when we get our nutrition from a variety of sources. And with good reason; life itself is full of variety!

I love eating according to the **15/6 rule**. My family and I live by this simple rule to make life easier. Typically, there are about 21 meals that we eat on a weekly basis; 7 breakfasts, 7 lunches, and 7 dinners. Basically, how this rule works is you eat at least 15 meals that are made at home. These meals should be made with whole, live, unprocessed foods (preferably organic and/or non-gmo) foods. Our motto is "If God made it, you're good to go. If man made it, RUN!" The other 6 remaining meals for the week can be enjoyed out with friends, family and so on because let's face it, "life" happens, and we aren't always able to eat at home. Following this strategy though, will make it easier for you to stick to your healthy lifestyle because you won't feel left out, you won't be missing anything, and you won't be feeling like you've "blown it'. So, go ahead, have your cake, and eat it too…just one piece is good though.

Speaking of cake! Oh, my sugar goodness! Who is not absolutely sugar-addicted? I believe the majority of us are! I know I am. I use the present tense because I have to be conscience of this every single day. Being mindful is in part, how I tackle my sugar cravings. The cravings do get weaker, but I feel if I don't keep my guard up, something is going to slip in there and send me into a downward spiral of chocolatey, gooey, sugary mess. Be sure to check out some of my recipes at the end of this book for some great craving-stopper, sugar substitutes.

There are functional medicine doctors who say this; if you're craving sweet treats, your body may really be needing more potassium. If you're craving chocolate, your body may really be needing magnesium. If you're craving starchy comfort foods, it may be that your body is needing more B vitamins. I think this is very interesting when we listen to our bodies and using strategic ways to curb our impulses may help.

Finding substitutions are a great strategy in my opinion. Here are some things I like to do to keep that sugar monster at bay. I like to make a delicious chocolate shake, that's actually healthy, early in the day to stop any sugar cravings that pop up. It's chocolate greens, and plant-based protein that I also add olive oil or Mct oil and cinnamon to, to make into a shake with either breakfast or lunch. It's satisfying because the protein and fat keeps you feeling fuller longer, and the chocolate goodness is sweetened with stevia. I feel like I'm getting a sweet treat!

Another thing I do when I'm really jonesing for sugar is to take a couple of squares of a Lily's chocolate bar, for example. We found this chocolate when my daughter had cancer and was on a strict no-sugar diet. Lily's chocolate is dark chocolate sweetened with stevia. They have a wonderful cancer story themselves and have several flavors of candy bars to choose from. They even have chocolate chips for healthier baking!

I keep frozen fruit like strawberries, bananas, blueberries, raspberries, and blackberries on hand to make some mind-blowing ice cream. Melt some of Lily's chocolate and pour it on top. Oh my! The options are endless and so dang delicious! If all else fails, I soak in a 40-minute Epsom salt bath. It is said that for the first 20 minutes of the bath, the salts pull out toxins from our body. I make it as hot as I can to really get a good sweat going for more detoxing effects. Then, for the next 20 minutes, our body pulls in the minerals of the Epsom salts by reverse osmosis. When you think about it, Epsom salts are high in magnesium. For me, I usually crave something chocolate. Dark chocolate is also a great source of magnesium. So, I'm actually craving magnesium, which most of us are deficient in anyway; not sugar! I can usually keep any thoughts of sweets away if I take just one Epsom salt bath a week!

Oh yes. Let's get back to talking about real food.

Real food is an integral part of total health. We need to raise the value of this statement. Real food is an integral part of total health! When we eat wholesome, unprocessed foods, there's really, little need to count calories. Now, of course, I'm not saying to eat a bushel of apples or three platefuls at dinner and you'll by fine! I only mean eat real, unprocessed food, and if you pay attention to how your body feels, your body will tell you when you've had enough to eat. This includes listening to our bodies for hunger pangs; true hunger pangs before we eat. Many of us just eat because it's lunch time or it's dinner time and we're really not hungry. It may be that we're just thirsty.

Which brings me to the subject of **water and liquids**. I usually tell my clients to drink half their body weight in ounces of filtered water every day, but I do realize that for some, this may be difficult. I think keeping our bodies sufficiently hydrated is what keeps our food digesting and metabolizing, keeps fluidity in our joints for better mobility, and keeps our kidneys and organs working properly. I love organic teas, especially green tea and green matcha tea. I do drink one cup of organic coffee every morning with one tablespoon of organic coconut oil, organic half and half, and a dash of cinnamon. I also try to steer clear of fruit juices because of the sugar content. If you're going to drink juices, make sure they are green juices, preferably that you make at home, and the very least, let them be organic juices. Drink them earlier in the day so that you burn off that sugar. I do love kombucha drinks and apple cider vinegar as well. If you're not familiar, these are fermented drinks that give our gut good probiotics (or healthy bacteria), which helps our immune system. Our gut is considered to be our "second brain" where 80% of our immune system is located, so it's not surprising that kombucha drinks are so beneficial for us.

The next time you eat, give this a try. Slow down and chew. Before you eat, take a deep breath or two and relax. Focus on the meal you are about to eat. Do your best to chew each bite at least 20 times and see how you feel. Chewing your food more completely greatly improves digestion and allows the body to be able to "read" the nutrients it was given. You'll find you feel fuller sooner, too, because the mind is able to read the stretch factor in the stomach. This one simple act at meal-time can make a really big difference in your health, as well as your weight-loss efforts.

Put an end to **snacking in between meals**. (Choose wisely if you must have a snack.) Snacking in between meals could be the cause to belly fat. In short, insulin is responsible for getting glucose from the bloodstream into muscle, fat and liver cells, where it can be used for ATP or energy, thereby lowering blood glucose levels.

Keep this in mind…every single time we eat, our pancreas shoots out insulin to gather up the sugar (glucose) in our blood. When we are eating too much, in this case it's snacking, the pancreas is unable to keep up and just shoots out more insulin. The muscle cells and liver cells then become resistant to the insulin; not allowing anymore in. so, because the insulin has to finish the job, it shoves it into the only cells that will allow it, and that is our fat cells. It's like a storage closet or attic that you just keep shoving more things in and hate the thought of clearing it out.

To help in keeping things in order, I recommend keeping a food journal. I know you've heard this before, but it really does make a difference. Even for the seasoned person who says they know what they are eating throughout the day. If you're having trouble anywhere in your health, keeping a food journal will help to open your eyes where the flaws are. Do more than just keeping track of what you eat. Write down when you eat, and how you feel when you're eating. Did you feel hunger pangs or just eat because it's scheduled? Did you get your water and liquids in or are you just thirsty? There's a lot we can record to gather the information we need to better our health. I challenge you to just give it a try.

I couldn't talk about diet without bringing up the "don't skip a meal" myth. I used to be guilty of this myself. By now, I'm sure you've heard of, or maybe even tried intermittent fasting. Intermittent fasting is when food is withheld for a period of hours, leaving another smaller period of hours in which to eat. So, typically, I recommend fasting for a period of 12 to 16 hours, leaving a window of 8 to 12 hours to eat. What some people don't realize, is that when we are sleeping, we are already fasting a period of at least 7 or more hours!

The benefits of fasting are many, but for the purpose of losing weight and controlling insulin resistance, I recommend doing a fast for 12 hours to start with. You would start counting the hours when you're done eating your last meal for the day. So, for example, you finished eating dinner by 6 p.m. You go to sleep for the night, wake up the next morning at 5 a.m. Get your morning rolling and before you know it, 6 a.m. is here and you've been fasting for 12 hours! You did it! See how easy that can be? When you get stronger and better at it, try to go 14 hours, then 16 hours, then 17 and 24 hours! Amazing things begin to happen inside our bodies after doing a 17 hour fast, for example. A process called autophagy happens. This is where our cells begin to clean up old and damaged cells throughout the body. This is defined as a process of self-digestion, meaning the body feeds upon itself!

The hormone ghrelin makes us used to eating at a certain time each day. Our bodies just love routine. You may need to do it a few times to adjust but I think you'll begin to find that your mornings will be more productive, your energy level will increase, and your metabolism will actually speed up. You may notice extra belly fat melting away. (This is meant for healthy people, but any concerns of any kind, consult with your physician before beginning fasting.) I also like to remind others that fasting is not just skipping meals. When meals are skipped, that means nutrition is also skipped and our body knows this. It will prepare for sparsity and slow down the metabolism. With fasting done right, a person will still get in the daily recommended nutrition when they do eat their meal.

Another important aspect that I love about fasting is the mindfulness that is required. You do have the ability to achieve your goals. Mindfulness, not will power, will do that and consistency is key.

The only thing left to discuss would be **supplements**. I won't get into all the different kinds of supplements there are because, quite frankly, there are just too many to discuss. I would rather just focus on some key points I learned. For specifics, because everyone is different and has different needs, I recommend you ask your medical provider or natural or functional medicine doctor.

I love supplements for many reasons. One main reason is that because of the use of so many gmo crops and farmers not rotating their fields, our soil has become very deficient in nutrients. This means that our foods are also deficient in these nutrients. With this in mind, I still recommend a food first approach, then supplement where needed. Don't just supplement for the sake of supplementing.

When choosing supplements to take, I make a very clear recommendation to read labels. It's best to get products with as many natural, non-gmo or organic, components as possible. I don't purchase any product with fillers or ingredients that are synthetic or chemical.

I also rotate the supplements my family and I use. As I mentioned before, our bodies become really efficient in our routines, so I change things up every couple of months. I'll also take breaks from using supplements. I was told by my functional medicine doctor that taking breaks from supplementation for about five to seven days, helps liver function.

Even though it's well-known that our soil in the U.S. is deficient, I still make reminders to get the nutrition from natural food sources first. Our bodies know this source first and foremost.

Chapter Four:
Exercise

Start moving! This is by far more important as we start reaching middle-aged life. Our bodies were meant to move, and you will hear me say this all the time. Honestly, you will feel more energy and less achy when you start even the smallest exercise routine. Exercise releases chemicals in our brain called endorphins, which makes us feel good. They trigger a positive effective in the body that's similar to morphine! These feel-good endorphins can help us to improve our mood.

Another extremely important reason to exercise is for muscle strength. We need to build and maintain muscle, especially as we age. Dr. Gabrielle Lyons says that skeletal muscle is our largest organ, not our skin. She says this is because muscle is more metabolically active.

This is what determines our health and quality of life. I, for one, want to see all of us more muscular as we age. I am working toward this myself.

Who's ready to work out now?

I remember one particular professor in college who told us we would serve ourselves well to exercise first thing in the morning before we start our day, because this gets those good chemicals pumping from the brain, boosting good hormones and releases much needed oxygen throughout our entire body, thus giving us more energy and more brain power for thinking the rest of the day. I'm not sure if he was just trying to stop people from sleeping in his class or if he meant to help, but I liked this advice. This makes more sense to me. Since I'm a morning person anyway, this works well for me.

Again, getting back to basics here, I always suggest three very simple exercises to start with that take up no space hardly at all, they're done quickly and require no equipment. It was my grandfather who taught me this routine, an elderly, retired Navy man who has long since passed away. It's just simple squats, simple push-ups, and regular ab crunches. Start off with 10-20 reps, for 1-3 sets. Work your way up to doing 25 reps for 4 sets. Try to add in a one-minute plank if you can.

Do whatever your fitness level allows at first and always take care of your joints. (Also check with your doctor if you need. Do not injure yourself by doing an exercise routine that may not be right for you at this time.) Feel free to add weights and resistance bands. Ladies, weights are your friend; don't be afraid to use them. I love doing this basic routine because it essentially works the entire body. It even gets a little cardio action going there. You can always add other exercises to this routine. Switching things up is good, as our bodies become really efficient when we have the same routine. It's very easy to switch up the technique used for push-ups, squats, and crunches as there are a variety of ways of doing them.

I love doing a Tabata type, HIIT (High Intensity Interval Training) or burst-type cardio workout and I recommend you try this if you haven't already. They're so powerful, that it is said the body will continue to burn fat, not sugar, for the next 24 to 48 hours, depending on how strong of a burst workout was performed. Let me tell you, when they say you will be burning for hours afterward, they mean you will be burning for hours afterward. I totally go through my own personal summer for the rest of the day! Rosie cheeks and all! I'm just sweating buckets! (So, plan your outfits accordingly ladies.)

There are plenty of YouTube videos out there to help you with this and they can be done in about 5 minutes. Seriously! Who doesn't like that? It's a serious workout in less time. No need for spending hours in the gym.

You must make time for exercise. Other active things you do throughout the day is wonderful, but you really need to set the intention to work out. You don't need hours to get this done, just a matter of a few minutes a day can make all the difference. Resting days in between workouts are vital, especially as we age. Here are some examples of workout routines.

Option 1:

Sunday: 30-minute brisk walk

Monday: 30-minute H.I.I.T. and stretches

Tuesday: 30-minute brisk walk

Wednesday: Strength training

Thursday: 30-minute brisk walk

Friday: 30-minute brisk walk

Saturday: 20-minute Strength training with 10-minute H.I.I.T.

Option 2:

Sunday: Rest

Monday: 30-minute brisk walk

Tuesday: Rest

Wednesday: 20-minute Strength training with
10-minute H.I.I.T.

Thursday: Rest

Friday: Strength training

Saturday: 30-minute brisk walk

Feel free to create a schedule around your daily routine. Keep this schedule for about 3-4 weeks, then change it up. Get creative and make it fun. Include the kiddos if you have them!

Stretching before and after your workouts are an important part to your whole routine, so don't leave this out. When we do a light stretch before we workout, this will increase our range of motion, flexibility, and circulation. All that good blood flow and oxygen gets into all your muscles and organs which will result in better performance and help to prevent injuries. Stretching after your workout allows the body to cool down. Blood circulation is returned to normal, allowing the heartbeat to return to normal also. When we workout, our bodies produce lactic acid. This is what makes the muscles feel sore and fatigued. When we stretch, that lactic acid is released and allows recovery and repair of the muscles. Typically, I say to take just two minutes before your workout to stretch and just five minutes after your workout. If you're doing a longer or harder level of exercise, adjust your stretching times to accommodate.

If you suffer from stiff shoulders, you may want to try this. Since I have had issues with stiff and frozen shoulders, I make it a point to stretch my shoulders before and after every workout I do. Stand by a door frame for example, hold the frame with one arm, then turn outward. So, your back is facing the door. Do this on each side. Everything we do is forward, like washing dishes, eating, writing, cleaning, picking things up from the floor. The muscles in the front of our shoulders never really get that good stretch because of this.

We all know that eating good foods with exercising regularly makes a big impact with our weight and overall health, but did you know about fasting? Combining exercise with fasting can provide wonderful benefits to your health as well. Performing exercises while being fasted has very impressive effects against insulin resistance, thus blocking sugar cravings. Once you get a good routine with fasting and exercising separately, maybe give the two of them together a try. (Please make sure with your doctor first. Fasting is not for everyone. We certainly don't want anyone injured or coming back saying that "I said to do this." This is just the practice that I do.)

There are more than just work-out routines to get in your exercise. Tennis anyone? Any sports activity does more than just burn calories. Swimming, bicycling, jogging, walking, basketball, volleyball, and yes, tennis; you get the idea. Keep in mind, also, our body is really efficient. I know I am repeating myself here. When we keep doing what we've always done, our body knows the routine and thus we are able to perform the action quite easily. Changing up your activities every once in a while, as we're reaching our midlife ages will help to protect us from diseases like Alzheimer's and dementia. So, get out there and try something new!

Have you tried rebounding? Rebounding is simply bouncing or jumping on a mini trampoline. I love rebounding! It makes me feel like a kid again. There are so many benefits to rebounding, I wasn't sure where to add this in the book! It's great exercise and a great detox, both of which are backed by NASA! You see, in the 1980's, NASA discovered rebounding when they needed an exercise that would reverse the damage to astronauts. They found that after being in zero gravity, astronauts would lose 15% of their bone and muscle mass. In short, NASA found that the entire body can be exercised with rebounding without an excessive amount of pressure to the feet and legs. There is less exertion on the heart but more benefit because of the increased G-force in rebounding, and it provides benefits on a cellular level that is better than exercises like running. Weight bearing exercises like rebounding increases bone mass. This becomes highly needed especially as we age.

Rebounding boosts lymphatic drainage. The detox part of this exercise comes in with the simple act of the up and down motion, which is highly beneficial for the lymphatic system because it runs in a vertical direction up and down the body. It does not have its own

pump to move lymph like the heart pumps
blood. The acceleration and deceleration of this
exercise causes each cell of the body to respond,
and since all cells are responding, it will increase
cellular energy and mitochondrial function.

I like to use my rebounder in between
sets of my workouts. It creates more of a high
intensity workout. I also use it if I'm feeling
tired or sluggish. Just two minutes gets the
oxygen moving and I'm feeling instantly more
energetic!

More benefits to rebounding include
boosting immune function, improves digestion,
improves balance by stimulating the vestibule of
the middle ear, improves oxygen circulation
throughout the entire body, improves muscle
tone, and some even say rebounding helps to
support the thyroid and adrenals! All this by just
having fun jumping up and down!

Chapter Five:

Getting Better Sleep and Reducing Stress

Getting better sleep sounds so dreamy, doesn't it? Like we must be forced to get this accomplished, but believe it or not, getting better sleep can be a difficult task for most of us. It's just the sign of the times, really. We live in such a fast-paced world, full of deadlines, egos, and unfinished business. It's just plain hard to relax!

Our body responds to stress, whether it is real or perceived, which means simply that our brain does not know the difference between what is real or fake. How we perceive something that is stressful or fearful, will determine if our brains signal chemicals dopamine, epinephrine, norepinephrine and if our adrenals secrete adrenaline and cortisol or not. These are what keeps us in the fight or flight mode. You know, when you get heated up, your heart starts racing and you feel tense all over? Cortisol raises our blood sugar which is not good in a constant state because this can lead to insulin resistance, a pre-diabetic state. When the stressful event is done, then our parasympathetic system kicks in to bring us back down to normal. Why is this important to know? Staying in the fight or flight mode for too long actually decreases our immune function and puts us at a higher risk for developing many different illnesses. Chronic stress can lead to more serious problems like heart disease, stroke, asthma, stomach ulcers, obesity, anxiety, depression, and panic attacks to name a few.

Stress management has a lot to do with getting better sleep and getting better sleep has a lot to do with stress management. Without enough sleep, our bodies feel the effects of stress much more than if we are rested. For both stress and better sleep, I am a lover of essential oils. Lavender is well-known for its relaxation properties, but have you heard about Magnesium Oil? I absolutely cannot be without these two together!

Magnesium is a water-soluble mineral that is needed for just about every process in our bodies! For this discussion, however, we'll keep it to how it helps us to relax and get better sleep.

Magnesium Oil Spray is actually not oil at all, but a highly concentrated mixture of filtered water and pure magnesium chloride flakes. Epsom salts are magnesium sulfate, which also promote good sleep. Magnesium chloride flakes are more usable by the body, which makes this the perfect ingredient for the Magnesium Oil Spray. This is called transdermal therapy, or through the skin, and it is absorbed very quickly into the bloodstream for maximum magnesium absorption.

My nightly routine consists of using my homemade Honey Hill Naturals (HHN) Lavender Fine Mist Spray. I use this spray on my pillow, sheets, and blankets. This makes a great natural sleep spray. I apply my HHN Magnesium Oil Spray on the bottoms of my feet. Then, I add lavender oil and maybe vanilla oil, or other relaxing blend in my oil diffuser near my bed. I can honestly say I sleep longer, more soundly and deeply when I use this routine for sleep.

When using this transdermal therapy for magnesium, there's no need to worry about overdosing since our bodies only take in what we need. It's a terrific supplement. Unlike when we take oral supplements, our bodies need to digest them and filter out the waste. Magnesium absorbs better through the skin than it does through the digestive tract. Epsom salt baths, magnesium lotions and gels are also great.

I have learned to reduce my stress by doing simple forms of meditating. I still find it difficult to do long meditations. I had to work up to even just doing ten to twenty minutes. It's very hard to quiet the mind when so much is going on but keep at it. The relaxation you get just from trying is beneficial itself. I have learned to let things go, especially things I have no control over. This was probably the hardest for me to do. Stress comes in many forms; life events, toxic people, money, and bills, etc. Be aware of your responses and acknowledge when you have to step out or take a break to care for your own wellness.

Like counting to ten, I have implemented using the mantra, *I love. I love. I love.* Christie Marie Sheldon on YouTube talks about her strategy of using this mantra to bring her energy to the level of love or above. I especially love using this method when people stress me out.

I found that staying away from sugar and processed foods was extremely helpful. Of course, comfort foods are comfort foods for a reason. Anything sugar-filled was my comfort food. I noticed very quickly that after eating my sugary comfort food, my knees and joints would ache, I would get a dull continuous headache, and stomach pains developed in the middle of the night, keeping me from a good night's sleep. So, I kept eating large salads even if I didn't feel like it, and green juices. All the chlorophyll-containing nutrition is wonderful for treating stress. Chapter seven has all the information on energies and emotions, which is useful with stress management and better sleep also.

Journal therapy is another powerful tool for destressing that I love! My daughter and I would use this natural therapy for so many areas in our life. Other ways to be proactive in stress management is by taking walks, bike riding, exercising or my favorite…just relaxing on the hammock. I bring a good book or magazine, some calming tunes and just be with nature under the trees. It is just so peaceful. My daughter would imagine sitting on the beach, listening to the waves crash against the shore. Nature itself is powerful against stress.

Grounding is where you walk around barefoot (in safe areas) to connect with the electromagnetic pull of the Earth. Many of us lost this totally by always being in rubber or plastic-soled shoes all the time. Walk along the beach and jump in the water. The effects of grounding alone will improve immune function, *sleep*, blood circulation, reduction of inflammation, reduce the effects of emf's, stabilize our body's basic biological rhythms and *reduce stress, anxiety, and irritability.*

I remember when I was a young mother, my favorite thing to do during the Spring and Summer months was to give my little ones a nice warm bath after a long day of playing and learning, dress them in some cute, comfy p.j.'s, pop them in the stroller and go for a nice long evening walk. It was so calming and destressing to me, and my babies would sleep so well all night long. I always credited that fresh air and nature. Time to get outside and play!

Chapter Six:
Reducing Toxicities

Reducing toxins involves the environment in your body as much as it involves the outside of your body. This includes your home, office space, planes or trains, and our vehicle. The truth of the matter is, whether you are aware or not, we are bombarded with so many toxins on a daily basis. It is reported that up to 300 man-made chemicals have been found to be in humans! I won't get into all of them but some of the more popular ones include pesticides, formaldehyde, mercury, antibiotics, fluoride, chlorine, benzene, lead, BPA, parabens, phthalates, copper, mercury, aluminum, ethanol, triclosan, hydrogenated oils, and high fructose corn syrup to name a few.

Quite a list already! These potentially harmful toxins are hidden in our foods, health care products, toiletries, kitchen plastics, and more.

If you need more help with learning all about toxins, label reading, products, symbols, and more, I can help you. There are numerous things to consider, and it can be quite overwhelming, to say the least. Many people don't even know where to begin. I offer a The Living Naturally Masterclass on my website that help you learn all of this information and more. *Find my website at the end of this book.

As I mentioned previously, one of my favorite articles is called *Cancer is a Preventable Disease that Requires Major Lifestyle Changes,* on PubMed. This article talks about how all the genes in our bodies have everything to do with environmental factors and exposure to toxins that will more likely determine if we get a disease than it does with "fate". It's very interesting. I encourage you to check it out.

The very weekend my daughter was diagnosed with cancer, we tore through the entire house getting rid of any household products that contained chemicals, and cooking utensils, pots and pans that were unsafe, and any food that was inorganic or basically processed. Needless to say, my house was bare. I know this is a costly move but so worth it in my opinion. According to the PubMed article I referred to in the previous paragraph, it says that pesticides may contribute to the cause of Ewing's Sarcoma. Now, of course we won't know the real answers until we meet the Big Guy, but you have to admit that a reliable source is letting us know the diseases these toxins may cause and how we can save ourselves from them.

Toxin exposure, especially of this magnitude, can lead to an increased risk of all sorts of chronic conditions and diseases. Also know that as bad as these toxins are to our bodies, they're just as toxic to the environment! So, if you're chronically ill, have MTHFR, or are dealing with a long-term diagnosis such as cancer, you may want to go through your own home and see what's lurking in your cupboards. I am certain you will be surprised how many chemicals and toxins are lying in wait.

Here is some of what I did. As I went through my home eliminating what I could, I got rid of my old non-stick pots and pans and traded them in for a tri-clad stainless-steel set. I disposed of all the plastic bowls and utensils and purchased glass, stainless-steel, or other BPA-free containers. (Use the least amount of plastics that you can. They're horrible for our us AND the environment! Plastics leach toxins into our foods and sit for hundreds of years in landfills. This includes water bottles, straws, and plastic bags.)

I replaced all pesticide-sprayed foods with organic ones. Never use a microwave oven. Use a toaster oven instead. And I no longer use store bought products for cleaning. Some people like to use essential oils when they clean. I just use a solution of 1/3 cup white vinegar, ¼ cup rubbing alcohol, and 3 cups filtered water in a spray bottle as my all-purpose cleaner. I use this everywhere and have had no issues with it. I like the way it cleans. In the bathroom, I use baking soda and white vinegar (be careful of the fizzy reaction). I sprinkle the baking soda in the sink and drain, around the tub and drain, and then in the toilet bowl. I then pour white vinegar over the baking soda. I think the fizzy action causes some of the cleaning power. I just use washable rags as well as my all-purpose cleaner to wipe all the surfaces down and its sparkling clean! I didn't have to purchase a bunch of chemical-filled products and my solution is also easy on the environment. I do purchase organic laundry detergent and dish soap, though. I did make my own for a time, but I found I just don't like it as well. I do not use toxic dryer sheets.

Of course, we want toxins to leave our body quickly. This is called detoxification. A great toxin reducer I like to use is a form of deep breathing. I do 4-7-8 breathing technique. Our body is naturally equipped with a built-in healing system, and deep breathing turns it on. Our lungs are one of the ways toxins are released from our body. Very simply, you inhale for 4 seconds. To be sure you are doing this correctly, your stomach and diaphragm should be filling first, pushing outward, then filling your chest. Then, hold your breath for a count of 7 seconds. This part of the exercise opens up the bottom of the lungs, called the dead space, where toxins lay in wait. Opening up more of your lungs moves those toxins out. Finally, release that breath slowly through your mouth for a count of 8 seconds, first emptying your chest, then diaphragm. Deep breathing is the switch that turns on to get that lymph moving. Rebounding can be your next step.

I spoke about all the great benefits of rebounding in the previous chapter. The up and down motions on a rebounder move the lymphatic system. Our lymph system is known as the garbage disposal of our body. The lymph fluid collects all the waste, cellular debris, cancer cells and toxins and removes them by dumping them into lymph nodes where they can be safely removed. Really, any form of exercise or movement will get the lymph fluid moving, but rebounding is a favorite in the natural therapy community because it does the job so efficiently and completely, and it has the endorsement by NASA. During my daughter's fight with cancer, one of the many treatments she used for detoxing her body was rebounding. When Tara wasn't able to jump on the rebounder, she would sit on the edge and bounce her bottom on the trampoline to get that same up and down motion as much as she could. You could even sit at the edge of your bed if your mattress is bouncy and get the same effect for that matter!

More great ways to detox is by drinking green juices, green smoothies, and eating lots of leafy green veggies, taking certain supplements like spirulina and chlorella, stimulating the liver by doing coffee enemas, dry brushing, sweating, hydrotherapy (which is switching from hot and cold water in the shower) and fasting. Fasting is something I love to do often. Intermittent fasting is something I do on an almost daily basis. When I was a Muslim, I also did a form of intermittent fasting in the form of full day, dry fasting. Eating plenty of fiber each day will naturally detoxify your body as well.

You may be more surprised to know that indoor air like in our homes and cars, are more toxic and chemical-filled than outdoor air! As much as ten times worse! These come from household products, cooking and heating, smoking, furniture and carpeting, mold, paints, and building materials. Of course, we can't eliminate all sources of these toxins, but we can use some natural solutions to create a more healthful environment.

Firstly, we can ventilate the rooms by opening windows as much as the weather will allow. I grew up in the Midwest and let me tell you, the long cold winter months did not stop my mother from airing out the house. She would bundle up my siblings and me in our snow-suits, full hats, scarves, and mittens, throw on some blankets and let us play on the floor while she opened up every window in the house to clear the air. I think it may have worked pretty well to release germs and toxins.

Other things we can do naturally is have plenty of house plants around. They breathe up all of our waste and give us clean oxygen to breathe in exchange. NASA stated, "Houseplants can purify and rejuvenate air within our houses and workplaces, safeguarding us from any side effects associated with prevalent toxins like ammonia, formaldehyde and also benzene."

I use lots of essential oils in all sorts of ways. I just love them! I have replaced using acetaminophen and ibuprofen products with peppermint and lavender oils, for example. I create my own immunity blends to wear on my body instead of wearing toxic perfumes. There are so many great companies out there now with great quality oils. Do your research. I use several brands. They don't have to be from only one company for you to enjoy the terrific benefits.

I love using Himalayan pink salt lamps and beeswax candles. Salt crystals work by pulling toxic water vapor out of the air as a natural ionic air purifier. The beeswax also ionizes the air and neutralizes toxins. Scented candles are usually a petroleum product and release lead and benzene into the air. If you can't replace your carpeting for a more organic one, the EPA says to take your shoes off at the door and use a doormat. This will reduce about 60% of toxins that are carried in by our shoes.

I also use activated charcoal in the form of bamboo. I have several of these bunches around, especially in my office where my computer is located as it loves to absorb all the electromagnetic (emf) waves. Charcoal bamboo carries a negative electric charge which attracts all the positively charged toxins.

I drink activated charcoal in my greens juices to help me detox once a month; it's also great to use when you get a case of food poisoning. Binders, such as activated charcoal and Shilajit (fulvic acid), for example, are quite beneficial when trying to detox as they bind, or stick to, the toxins and then we just release it through our urine or poop. Shilajit is said to be especially helpful with a toxic load of heavy metals.

I make my own organic activated charcoal soap for the shower, and I also brush my teeth with it. It's a great teeth whitener as it cleans!

On the subject of EMF's; these are also a very dangerous indoor air pollutant. You can do things like turning your Wi-Fi off at night, turn off computers, routers, and printers while you sleep, and use TV's and computers that have LCD screens instead of plasma screens. You can find so many articles on emf's and ways to reduce them in your home and office. I think do what's best for you and your family. There are many easy ways to lower emf exposure. I, myself, did purchase emf safety blockers for our cell phones. I cringe when I see someone giving a small child a cell phone to play with. It's just not a good idea. I use an aluminum baking sheet underneath my laptop, although they do make pads for this that are much more aesthetically pleasing. I think about all those teens who have to put their laptop right on their thighs near their reproductive organs. I turn off lights when I'm not using them, and I don't even know how many years it's been since I've even touched a microwave oven! There really is so much more you can easily do to protect you and your family.

I am aware that some risk to being exposed to toxins is unavoidable but reducing your total body burden of toxins will help out tremendously. Practicing a toxic and chemical-free lifestyle is easier than you may think. What are some ways you can reduce toxin levels or chemicals in and around your home and body

today? Give it a try!

Chapter Seven:
Master Your Emotions/Energy

Aaaahhh. Emotions and energy. We certainly are emotional beings, aren't we? I almost wanted to lump stress and emotions together, but I think it may be better to manage them apart from each other, even though our emotions can cause us great stress at times. In my experience, working on them separately and one at a time gave me much more power within myself to heal.

Everything in this world is made up of energy. Did you know a rock has energy? Yes, even inanimate objects have energy. Energy is what gives our body physical mass. Okay, I'm not a physicist but I do a lot of research. Did you know that emotional energy is what gives rise to metaphysical conditions in our body?

What does metaphysical mean anyway? Well, metaphysical pertains to metaphysics, and just like we know how physics deals with laws that regulate the physical world, metaphysics deals with what is beyond the physical. *Metaphysics* comes from the combination of two Greek words; *meta*, meaning over and beyond, and *physics*, which means over and beyond physics. It is a huge area of study. The way I simplify it for my thinking, is that it is having to do with all the energy of "true" reality (not just what we perceive), that's beyond the physical plane (and beyond our physical selves. So, in my humble opinion, our emotions and core beliefs will manifest ailments in our physical bodies from the energy we give out; and knowing this will also help us to heal from these ailments. This, to me, is why conventional medicine doesn't always work on pains and symptoms when no injury was had. The pains are stemming from our emotional body.

We know that emotions are real, right? We feel them, that's for sure. Each of us goes through emotional trauma. It's just a fact of life.

Emotions, though, are really energy that manifests into our bodies that cannot be seen or even measured in any tangible way. Western medicine has devalued our emotions as far as contributing to any ailments we may create in our bodies. I, for one, am living proof of the metaphysical health I have created. By this I mean, for instance, when my only daughter was dying from cancer, I began experiencing pain in my knee, shoulder, and neck in the few months prior to her passing. I remember telling her doctor as we sat in the pediatric oncology clinic, that I felt like I was having sympathy pains for my daughter. To which she replied, "That's a very real thing."

As, I began to heal my body, I literally used everything I have mentioned in this book. As they say, when there is a fire burning out of control, you call in the fire department, you bring in the hose from outside, you get your neighbors hose, and so on. You gather everything you can to put out that fire! You hit from every angle. When it came to be having to deal with my energy and emotions, this took everything I could give. Understand that I feel I am empathic. I believe I actually work through things pretty thoroughly and quickly, and I believe my age allows me to be older and wiser these days. I know my body very well.

So, on with it; this is what I did. With me, all things are based on the belief that there is only one true creator. (I am Muslim, so I call my creator Allah. It's totally fine whatever your beliefs are.) With this belief, I believe that my body has a right over me. That means it has the right to be healthy; fed good nourishment, be physically fit, emotionally fit, spiritually, and mentally fit. It's all connected. I believe all that I do is in worship to my creator, so I try to begin all things with some sort of prayer. My point being, lean into your religion and faith.

My next steps were that I began working on my energy. I felt this needed to be done before I tackled my emotions. Emotions to me seem so half-hazard at times and it's easier to check where that energy is coming from. Have you ever tried qigong? Yoga may work well for this also; however, my physical body was in such a state of pain that I could no longer do yoga. It caused me a great deal of stress. I found that qigong was something that allowed me to focus only on my energy and it taught me great control of it while I was healing the soreness of my body. I encourage you to give this a try if you haven't done it before. I felt so amazing after my first session I can't even tell you! I felt less depressed on those days and my (physical) energy was sustained for the entire day, which is difficult to do when you have chronic fatigue syndrome. Keep up this practice. It is amazing for you.

As I kept with this practice of managing my energy, I found I was soon able to focus on clearing bad energy, or energy blocks from me. Whether it was from the stress of loss or having to deal with toxic people, I was able to clear that bad negative feeling. I recognized that I could focus on the feeling it gave me. So, for example, I would get stomach pains instantly from this bad energy. I would say my prayer or give myself a blessing and then literally take my hand over my stomach and act as if I was pulling out this ball of bad energy. Then I would throw it away from me, like I was throwing it out. Strangely enough I have to admit, the pain was instantly gone, and I felt this "good feeling" come over me. My mother always said use the power of your mind, so whether or not this is all just in my head, I choose to have the power. Give it a try and see if this works for you.

Emotions, then, were easier for me to manage after I was able to handle my energy. If I was feeling sad or depressed, I would think about and imagine things that made me feel good, joy, or happiness. If I was angry, I was able to logically look at what made me angry

and think of all the different ways I could react.
Doing this made it easier for me to see that an
outburst or temper tantrum wasn't the best
reaction for every situation. I'm human, though,
so I'm far from perfect, but this helped me to
feel one hundred percent better about my
situations in life and to start creating the things
I wanted to do to make me happier.

Chapter Eight:

Informed Conventional Care, Products   I Love, and Natural Remedies

There's a time and place for conventional medicine. If I am in an emergency situation, believe me! I want all the things and all the drugs to stop my pain! I don't want a Reiki master waving lavender over me. Well, maybe afterward I do, but not during the actual emergency.

In a perfect world, conventional will be combined with natural therapies, and if you can find a practitioner who is willing to do that, consider yourself lucky! Throughout my entire health journey to holistic living, I have had all sorts of reactions from people and medical doctors alike. Of course, I love learning with the ones who already live this way. They taught me so much. I've met so many that, in turn, were eager like myself and learned from me. And even though there is so much proof that our bodies respond so well to natural therapies, I get those people and doctors, that attack me, thinking that I'm totally against conventional western medicine. I think I've had just about every reaction!

The truth is, I'm not totally against it; conventional medicine that is. I only believe we should be more attuned to our own health and well-being and not depend on a pill to make things right, is all. Integrative, or natural, medicine treats the cause of a disease or ailment and is something that honors the body's own innate wisdom and ability to heal itself; by treating the body as a whole and uses all available therapies. Conventional medicine treats the disease or ailment, not the cause and uses information based on scientific evidence, though many of the tests are skewed by the people who fund them to get the results that they want. Conventional care in my opinion, is most useful in emergent situations for example. When you break your ankle skiing or fall in the shower breaking your wrist and need to have the bones surgically set or get a deep cut while slicing food and need stitches for it to heal, or have a heart attack, or get into a car accident, or…. see the trend? It uses drug-based, chemical medicines that are fast or faster acting than many natural treatments, which of course offers faster relief. In all of the healing processes though, it is the body that actually heals itself. The doctor can set the bone in the right place and cast it, pin it, or staple it together. It is the body that mends the broken bones or skin tissue back to health, in whatever form that may be.

There are a few natural items I hope I won't ever be without in my natural medicine cabinet. They are essential oils like peppermint, lavender, lemon, and frankincense, activated charcoal, vinegar or apple cider vinegar and oil of oregano. Good old-fashioned Himalayan or sea salt, too!

Here are some great examples of how I use some natural therapies. I share these with you to show ways in which I take care of myself. In no way am I implying that you do not seek the advice of your doctor for any reason whatsoever.

I love using essential oils! You'll hear me say this often. If you haven't tried them before but were interested, I always suggest starting with maybe three oils; lavender for better sleep and relaxation, peppermint for natural relief of headaches and body aches, and lemon or lemongrass for cleansing or refreshing. Two bonus oils would be Frankincense or Tea Tree oils for their many medicinal properties that are reported. I use peppermint oil (directly or with a carrier oil) for headaches. I haven't used NSAID's in years. I use peppermint and lavender together with a carrier oil like jojoba oil to relieve pain and inflammation on muscles and joints. I no longer use topicals like Ben-Gay or Flexall. I use essential oils and carrier oils to make my own chest rub, all-purpose healing creams, and daily moisturizers. I have replaced all other lotions, creams, and soaps with my own handmade products. (i.e., no chemicals.) I replaced heavy scented perfumes with my own essential oil sprays and roll-ons. Not only are these more pleasing to strangers than heavy perfumes, but these oils are building my immune system at the same time. I use Tea Tree oil to get rid of nail fungus, the itch from mosquito bites, as well as mixed with one of my creamy salves to relive eye styes and other skin infections. It's great for acne too!

I use activated charcoal for numerous things like whitening my teeth, or drinking it mixed with water for a monthly detox, and this works very well if you get food poisoning! I also use it in my own handmade soaps.

My daughter cured her candida infection in her gut using oil of oregano (nature's antibiotic) with the guidance of her natural doctor. Conventional medicine would have prescribed some form of antifungal or antibiotics to treat this that may not have even been successful. (My daughter was so successful with this treatment in part because she cut out ALL sugar from her diet, and I do mean all.) I cured many staph infections on myself using oil of oregano, but there were infections that my daughter and I needed conventional antibiotics for, especially when her immune system was impaired by chemotherapy. Another incident with my daughter's tumor wound; the wound nurse at the hospital knew how much my daughter wanted to use natural products as much as possible, so she gave us Medihoney. Knowing all too well the benefits of honey and wound healing, we quickly fell in love with it.

I love using pink Himalayan sea salt for various things. Of course, I think we all know about the gargling with warm salt water for getting rid of a bothersome sore throat. I also use the pink salt in a mixture with baking soda to clean my teeth, along with iodine. I use it as a solution in my water-pic machine. (My next health adventure by the way, is healing my teeth naturally.) Natural dentists say this helps to keep away all those swimming "bad bugs" in your mouth! I've used pink salt solution in warm water to help heal eye styes as well. It has worked wonders for me! I also take some key supplements for healing my teeth and they are vitamin D3 (at least 5,000 IU's), emo oil (cod liver oil if you're not allergic to fish like I am), and grass-fed butter oil. These nutrients are key for teeth.

I had used black salve from the Amazon rain forest to heal a presumed skin cancer spot on my chest, over my collarbone. After my daughter had passed away from her cancer, I went back to work right away. I have a medical billing office background and one day, while I was picking up the weekly billing from one of our providers, the doctor's wife (who also happens to be a doctor) stopped midsentence to tell me that the mole on my collarbone looked like skin cancer. I don't have to tell you that my stomach did a flip. She proceeded to explain that in her opinion, it appeared to be melanoma. She asked me a few questions about it. It was about the size of a pencil eraser. Well, I brushed it off temporarily to regain my composure with the whole thought of having to deal with cancer once again. I did a lot of research and came across black salve. I spoke with natural doctors in the past about using this stuff with my daughter, so I was well aware of the product.

It only works on cancerous cells and will not hurt normal skin cells, so I thought why not give it a try? I know what conventional medicine will do to me and it is always there if I need it. I was ready to try it for myself. (I am not recommending you try black salve for yourself. I am not recommending you should not see your doctor. Take care of yourself. I am only telling a story of what I did for myself.) I ordered the black salve and the dragon's blood product together for $30.00. It took one week, and the skin cancer fell out into my band-aid. It took another week and the hole left in my skin was now soft, new pink skin in its place. I was super amazed! During this time, I also did other things like drank green juices every day, did rebounding to clear my lymph system, took some key supplements like turmeric and flax seed oil, ate lots of big salads and fruits and veggies galore! Of course, I also stayed away from anything sugary or processed.

I am somewhat fair-skinned; however, I do tan for being so fair and I can hold a tan for quite a while. I have had hundreds of sunburns though, especially there on my chest, so I will take care to use a very good, organic sun-block from now on. Regular suntan or sunblock lotions may actually cause cancer as they are filled with chemicals like oxybenzone, avobenzone, octisalate, octocrylene, retinyl palmitate, homosalate and octinoxate. Be well-informed and do your research when going out in the sun. Sun is good for you; it is the best source of vitamin D. Just don't be out in it for too long or burn for your skin type. If you're having to deal with a cancer diagnosis, I urge you to check out www.cancertutor.com. This website has so much information on healing all types and stages of cancer, by using mostly natural means!

I believe in using chiropractic care to set my spine into alignment, allowing for proper nerve function and blood flow to all organs and joints. Chiropractic care has taken away the many joint pains that I was suffering from in my neck, shoulder, hips and lower back, knees, and ankles, which were not caused by any injury. I had frozen shoulder on my left side (amongst other joint pain issues) that greatly limited my range of motion. My frozen shoulder was pushing my collar bone out forward, my scapula was protruding outward, and my spine was twisting a bit. The muscles that run up and down my thoracic spine was very short and tight as well, from not using my left shoulder. It's amazing how so much is connected. I could barely move properly. Even doing everyday things like getting dressed and showering were quite difficult. I was in so much pain and my arm was beginning to lose function. I couldn't pull open a door with my left arm. The nerve would shoot pain all of a sudden and I would drop whatever I was carrying.

I received spinal adjustments, physical therapy, acupuncture, therapeutic massage, ultrasound, electrical stimulation, and infrared sauna therapy while at the chiropractic office. Within a month I was feeling so much better. I was able to function better and had less pain very rapidly. Within four months, my arm was moving to 160-degree range of motion with ease. And still today, my arm continues to improve and get stronger with almost full-range of motion.

Inquiry reduces fear when it comes to any health treatment, whether it is conventional or holistic. Overall, the goal is quality of life. Ask tons of questions while you're seeking knowledge. Hold yourself accountable for your health. My point is, take care of yourself. Learn to eat for living a healthy life; not living to eat. Eat well; eat a variety. Move more instead of planting yourself in front of the television set. Find balance. This is the only body we have been given. We only get one. We need to do our best to take care of it, no matter what age we are. Do things at your own pace and what's best for your body and your family. If you don't want to live off the grid, then don't! Go somewhere in between that you like. Any little change makes big improvements overall.

Collectively, we have to stop looking for ways to make our health "more convenient". It's just not working this way. It's not about convenience in my opinion.

Bonus Information – Natural Biohacks to Lower Glucose Spikes, Crashes, and Insulin Levels

Insulin Resistance, Diabetes type 2, hypertension, and other diseases are a choice that we make that is centered completely around the foods we choose to eat. We must remember that sweet foods were intended to be for our pleasure, not to be centered around.

*The Glucose Goddess, Jesse Inchauspe, a biochemist, did a deep dive into these biohacks that have been around for a very long time and put them all together in her book. Be sure to check that out. A big thank you to her for helping out us health coaches with this useful information! With that, let's get right into the biohacks.

Start your day by eating a (Keto) Savory Breakfast

The typical American diet usually includes very sweet meal choices, like pancakes and syrup, waffles with more syrup with sweet cream sometimes, fruits, oatmeal, cereals, etc. Try eating a savory breakfast, such as veggies and eggs. This would look like two radishes chopped with one quarter zucchini chopped, and maybe some peppers, with three eggs scrambled with a handful of chopped spinach and garlic with salt and pepper to taste. Top this all off with some real butter and even a little sprinkle of cheese. This savory breakfast provides us with less insulin release which means no glucose crash. Our hunger hormones are more steadied, and we crave less. This is the epitome of a ketogenic meal.

Link to study

https://pubmed.ncbi.nlm.nih.gov/30968140/

(Keto) Apple Cider Vinegar (ACV) Drink

The very basic ACV drink is to start out with 1 tablespoon of acv in an 8 to 10 oz glass of filtered water. This can be consumed any time throughout the day,(1 to 3 times per day before meals is fine) but to lower a glucose spike and crash from food, drink this before your meal.

Keto drink (Vinegar Mocktail) – This is my version of a Vinegar Mocktail. Make ahead of time some green tea, chilled. You can sweeten this with stevia if you'd like. Any glass you're using, fill the glass at least half full of ice. Pour about 1/4th cup (or 1 to 2 shot glasses full) of organic apple cider vinegar with the mother, add prepared green tea to fill the glass half way, then top it off with San Pellegrino mineral water. The mineral water is slightly carbonated making this drink look super festive. Add a dash of salt. Stir slightly to mix. Only drink this one or two times a day and it is recommended to drink with a straw to save from the acid wearing away at the enamel on your teeth. I have also read that because the ACV is diluted with water, your teeth should be fine. I'm not totally sure about this so just take precaution. Discontinue if stomach upset occurs.

Food Order

Eat your veggies before your (starchy) meal. Eat your veggies first, then fats and proteins, and finally, starchy foods and sugary foods last. This will cut the glucose spike by 73%. It's okay to eat them all together if the foods are mixed.

What this does is the fiber creates a fibrous mesh within the gut lining which sort of "catches" the other foods that come after it. This slows down the digestion and thus, slows down the sugar spike.

Link to Study

https://pubmed.ncbi.nlm.nih.gov/30101510/

Movement after eating

Incorporate some movement after eating to bring down insulin resistance. This can be getting up to wash your dishes, do some laundry, fold the clothes, clean a room, declutter an area, etc. Walking is the best movements you can do after your meal.

https://www.ncbi.nlm.nih.gov/pmc/articles/PMC8912639/

Resistant Starches

Resistant starches are a type of glucose found in grains, potatoes, and rices. They can be good for us because they also function much like soluble fiber. "Some of its potential benefits include improved insulin sensitivity, lower blood sugar levels, reduced appetite, and various benefits for digestion." One type in particular is my second tip here today. This starch "Is formed when certain starchy foods, including potatoes and rice, are cooked, and then cooled. The cooling turns some of the digestible starches into resistant starches via retrogradation." My tip then, when eating rice, potatoes, or pasta, make your plate with portion size in mind and let it cool down. This should help to lower blood sugar spikes, and thus help with weight loss.

This tip is often not supported by the medical field; however, the Glucose Goddess has shown this to be true as far as her blood glucose monitor. I would recommend testing this out for yourself.

Dress your Foods

Add healthy fats to your carbs to help slow down the glucose response, much like in the food order. This would be real butter and/or sour cream on your baked potato with the skin on, or nut butter to your cracker or apple slice.

Soleus Muscle Pushups

The Soleus muscle was discovered by scientists at the University of Houston. This muscle was found to specifically reduce glucose spike after a meal, all from the comfort of your chair! The soleus is found in the calf muscle, underneath the gastrocnemius muscle. It is the main muscle responsible for standing, walking, and running. This muscle is quite amazing as it never gets tired. This means you can keep using this muscle to soak up the circulating glucose to use for energy after your meal. Try to do this for ten minutes (or more) after your meal.

Link to Study

https://pubmed.ncbi.nlm.nih.gov/36034224/

Fasting and MCT Oil

Fasting

We were never meant to be grazing on food all day long. We are not cows. We also were not meant to be fasting every day. I believe in variety and circadian rhythm, so with that, I believe it's best to mix things up overall. When beginning to fast, I recommend build up your time restrained eating or intermittent fasting on a 16/8 schedule to start with. (Do not fast if you are pregnant, trying to get pregnant, or nursing.) Try closing in your eating hours to only 8 hours during the day. I recommend keeping this window open more to the daylight hours ending anywhere between 3 and 5 pm, not ending in the evening. Eating during the daylight hours works more in tandem with our cortisol hormones, the dawn phenomenon, and our sleep/wake cycle (our circadian rhythm). The fasting hours provides a better environment for your digestion to "rest" without having to process and metabolize foods. It will promote better bowel flow and better sleep. You can drink fluids like water, mineral water, teas, black coffee, and apple cider vinegar during the fasting time. It is recommended to stay hydrated for best intestinal flow.

During the time of the eating window, do not worry about counting calories at this time. Remain mindful of the amount you are eating, though. I recommend keeping a journal for this. Focus on three meals with no snacks. If you must eat a snack, try to make it one of the healthy fat choices so limit the rise in insulin. We want to allow the body more time to digest. Longer fasts will come later when your body is fat-adapted, meaning able to handle the fasts on a healthy level.

*Dr. Mindy Pelz has some amazingly helpful information on all things fasting. She has written several books, with her latest book called Fast Like a Girl. Be sure to check this out.

Link to study for 16/8 fasting

https://www.sciencedaily.com/releases/2018/0 6/180618113038.htm

<u>Mct Oil</u>

Mct oil is the perfect fat, especially for someone without a gallbladder. This type of fat does not get digested. This fat literally gets absorbed right into the liver and forces the liver to make ketones. This is a great source of clean energy for the whole day.

MCT's also offer heightened immune support and even weight loss. Mct is short for medium-chain triglycerides, specifically C8 (caprylic acid) and C10 (capric acid). MCT's are known to be in coconut oil, however, the C8 and C10 acids are named after goats. "Additionally, caprylic acid is found naturally in the breast milk of certain mammals like humans and goats. As a matter of fact, the Latin word for goat, Capra, is the root of caprylic acid!"

Links

https://naturalforce.com/blogs/nutrition/c8-c10-c12-medium-chain-triglycerides

https://naturalforce.com/blogs/nutrition/capr
ylic-acid

Grounding

Grounding or earthing is a term we use in the
natural world for going outside and touching
some part of nature with our physical body.
This means to take your shoes off and walk in
the grass, the dirt, the sand, or the water. It
doesn't matter which. Touch a tree. Run your
fingers across the blades of grass. The earth
literally reconnects us and discharges us of the
bad energies we collect in our tissues.
According to Jesse Inchauspe, a study from
Poland shows that grounding can also improve
glucose levels. It is thought to work by reducing
our stress levels much like sports, hobbies, or
relaxation activities, which directly impacts our
glucose levels. Grounding is thought to reduce
inflammation in the body by providing
electrons of the magnetic field of the earth,

which this may indirectly improve glucose levels as well.

So, go smell all the roses and hug all the trees!

Link to study

https://pubmed.ncbi.nlm.nih.gov/21469913/

It's well known that, unfortunately, doctors are not taught very much at all concerning healthy nutrition. They are trained by Big Pharma (and probably also Big Food). This means they are taught about medicines, not foods. This is where holistic nutritionists and health coaches come in. We deep dive into nutrition every single day. We know the ins and outs of nutrition that doctors just do not. Reversing is a long, slow, almost painful process to reverse, but it can be done! Problems with insulin begin decades before resistance is noticed.

Chapter Nine:
Recipes and Substitutions

I hope you find the following recipes and substitutions tasty and helpful. They are my most favorite that I use daily for me and my family. I do not have any nutritional value listed, as these are just recipes I use. I always try to use only organic, non-gmo food choices to get the best nutritional worth that I can. You may be able to plug the ingredients into an app or FitBit to get nutritional values that way. I love the Food Data website that gives very specific nutrient information that you plug in to get your own chart of results. Very handy resource!

Also, any of these recipes are very forgiving and ingredients can be easily interchangeable. Like potatoes in the Lentil Soup can be switched out with cauliflower or the pasta in the Veggie (Chicken) Soup can be swapped with zoodles for lower carb options. Either way… Enjoy!

Smoothies and Drinks I Love

One of my favorite ways to get in lots of good veggies with high amounts of nutrition is by making one of these green smoothies.

Build a Green Smoothie

1. **Choose your base, 2 cups of your choice**
    a. Filtered water
    b. (Cold) Green Tea, steeped in fridge
    c. Nut milk
    d. Raw coconut water
2. **Choose your fruit, fresh or frozen**
    a. ½ Avocado
    b. ½ cup Blueberries
    c. Banana
    d. ½ Green apple, chopped
3. **Choose your leafy greens, 2 large handfuls (2 cups)**
    a. Spring mix
    b. Romaine
    c. Kale
    d. Swiss chard
    e. Bok choy
    f. Dandelion
    g. Spinach
    h. Parsley
    i. Beet tops

4. **Choose Protein**
    a. Whey, grass-fed protein powder
    b. Plant protein, pea protein
    c. Bone broth or collagen powder
5. **Optional boosters**
    a. 1 tbsp Chia seeds
    b. 1-2 tsp Spirulina
    c. 1-2 tsp Cracked cell Chlorella
    d. 1-2 tbsp Flaxseed, ground
    e. 1-2 tbsp MCT oil
    f. 1-2 Packets of Stevia or Monk Fruit
    g. 1-2 tsp Cinnamon
6. **Blend and enjoy!**

Green chocolate protein smoothie – Use a high-powered blender for best results. I use a Ninja blender.

Ingredients and Directions:

200 oz. filtered water

2-3 (packed) cups greens like kale or baby kale, spinach, celery (cut up in 3-inch pieces), beet tops, Swiss chard, romaine, or greens of your choice.

Blend until greens are completely chopped and blended together.

Add 1 cup unsweetened almond milk (optional)

1 ripe banana

½ avocado

Serving of protein powder according to package instructions. (I use an organic plant-based protein powder.)

2 tablespoons organic cocoa powder

1-2 tablespoons raw organic honey or dates for sweetness (optional)

Dash of cinnamon (optional)

4 ice cubes

Blend until all is completely mixed well. Then, enjoy! All those fruits and veggies in one powerful, healthy drink! I drink this in the mornings for breakfast when I'm not fasting. It keeps me energized and satisfied for hours until lunch!

Green berries protein smoothie – Use a high-powered blender for best results. I use a Ninja blender.

Ingredients and Directions:

200 oz. filtered water

2-3 (packed) cups greens like kale or baby kale, spinach, celery (cut up in 3-inch pieces), beet tops, Swiss chard, romaine, or greens of your choice.

Blend until greens are completely chopped and blended together.

Add 1 cup unsweetened almond milk (optional)

1 small apple

½ avocado

Serving of protein powder according to package instructions. (I use an organic plant-based protein powder.)

1 cup berries (Can be frozen or fresh. I use strawberries, black berries, raspberries, and blue berries.)

1-2 tablespoons raw organic honey or dates for sweetness (optional)

Dash of cinnamon (optional)

4 ice cubes

Blend until all is completely mixed well. This shake definitely fixes my sweet tooth! Enjoy!

Green Tea Flush

I make two large jars or pitchers of iced organic green tea. I will drink this for one entire day to flush out my liver and kidneys. You must use filtered or clean water with organic green tea bags. You may have your morning coffee and drink water throughout the day as long as you can finish the green tea for the flush.

Keto ACV Drink

Make ahead of time some green tea, chilled. You can sweeten this with stevia if you'd like. Any glass you're using, fill the glass at least half full of ice. Pour about 1/4th cup (or 1 to 2 shot glasses full) of organic apple cider vinegar with the mother, add prepared green tea to fill the glass half way, then top it off with San Pellegrino mineral water. The mineral water is slightly carbonated making this drink look super festive. Add a dash of salt. Stir slightly to mix. Only drink this one or two times a day, preferably before meals. Discontinue if stomach upset occurs.

Lemon Ginger Shots

Firstly, some info on ginger. Ginger root is a well-known spice that has been longed used in cooking as well as medicine. Did you know that it is closely related to turmeric and cardamom? It contains antioxidant properties and some

very powerful compounds called "gingerols",
"shogaol", "paradol", and "zingerone". These
compounds help greatly to bring down
inflammation in our bodies.

Inflammation increases our risk for diseases like
cancer and chronic illnesses.
Ginger boosts our immunity and can quickly
relieve symptoms from the flu, cold and
respiratory viruses.
Ginger aids in digestion as well as helps to treat
many forms of nausea.
Ginger can help to lower blood sugar levels and
may even help with weight loss.
And there's so much more!! Ginger can be
enjoyed in so many ways, whether it be raw,
cooked, dried, as an oil, or powdered in a
capsule. It can be ingested or used topically on
the body. I slice it and add it to my teas.

Here's the recipe I use for the shots.

Ingredients:

1 palm size ginger root, chopped into chunks

2 small to medium lemons (or one large one), chopped into pieces

¼ teaspoon ground Turmeric

Dash of black pepper

2 tablespoons honey

Extra Items Needed:

2-quart bowl and flour sack towel for straining mixture

Instructions:

Place ginger root and lemon pieces (skins and all) into high powered blender. Blend until completely pulverized together. Pour into the bowl with the flour sack towel. Pick up all four corners of the towel together, catching the sides and twist. Keep twisting to strain the mixture into the bowl. The pulp left over can be discarded or added to your compost heap.

I then pour the juiced part into my Ninja bullet to further mix the remaining ingredients. You can use another mixer or hand mixer if you'd like. Add in the turmeric, pepper, and honey. Give it a good mix to thoroughly blend.

Store in the refrigerator for up to one week. (This tastes a whole lot better when cold.) This drink is very spicy so don't let it catch you off guard. Keep a chaser of water available if you need it. Take a 2 to 4 ounce shot every morning before eating breakfast.

This can taste very hot and spicy, so be careful. Let me know how you like it!

Beet Shots

Ingredients:

2 to 3 beets, chopped into chunks

1 thumb-size ginger root, chopped into chunks

1 lemon chopped into pieces, skin, seeds, and all

¼ teaspoon ground Turmeric

Dash of black pepper

2 tablespoons honey

Extra Items Needed:

2-quart bowl and flour sack towel for straining mixture

Instructions:

Place all ingredients into a high powered blender. Blend until completely pulverized together. Pour into the bowl with the flour sack towel. Pick up all four corners of the towel together, catching the sides and twist. Keep twisting to strain the mixture into the bowl. The pulp left over can be discarded or added to your compost heap.

I then pour the juiced part into my Ninja bullet to further mix the remaining ingredients. You can use another mixer or hand mixer if you'd like. Add in the turmeric, pepper, and honey. Give it a good mix to thoroughly blend.

Store in the refrigerator for up to one week. (This tastes a whole lot better when cold.) Take a 2 to 4 ounce shot every morning before eating breakfast and lunch.

Breakfasts

Chia Seed Pudding (also good as a snack)

Overnight Chia Pudding – high in omega 3 and healthy fats. Makes a great swap for something sweet.

Refrigerated

3/4 cup Almond milk, unsweetened

1/4 cup heavy whipping cream

Condiments

1-2 packets Stevia or Monk Fruit to taste

Baking & Spices

1 tsp Vanilla extract, pure

Nuts & Seeds

3 tbsp Chia seeds

1 tbsp flaxseeds, ground, optional

Toppings

Blueberries

Coconut flakes

.

Pro Tip: Blend in a high speed blender to really get the mixture blended well. This helps greatly with the texture issue as it is so much smoother!

Keto Treat

Makes a great type of "cereal" or a swap for something sweet.

Ingredients:

½ cup heavy whipping cream or coconut cream (in a can)

1 Stevia packet, then eventually no sweetener

Mix-ins/Toppings:

Blueberries

Crushed walnuts

Chia seeds

Directions:

Use a hand mixer to fluff up the heavy whipping cream. If you're using the coconut cream, you may not need to do this step. That's it! This makes two servings. Set in bowls and refrigerate. This can be chilled for a while or eaten right away. Add in your toppings when ready to eat.

Soups and Chili

Lentil Soup

Total Time: 50 min

Ingredients:

1 pound organic grass-fed ground beef (or meat of your choice)

2 tablespoons organic extra virgin olive oil or coconut oil, plus extra for drizzling

1 organic medium onion, chopped

2 organic carrots, peeled and chopped

2 organic celery stalks, chopped

2 organic garlic gloves, chopped

Organic Sea Salt and pepper to taste

1 diced organic tomato

2 handfuls organic baby spinach leaves

1 ¼ cups organic lentils

11 cups organic chicken broth

1 tablespoon organic Italian seasoning

6 organic potatoes, chopped

1 cup Parmesan cheese

Directions:

Brown ground beef, drain and set aside.

Heat the oil in a heavy large pot over medium heat. Add the onion, carrots, and celery. Add the garlic, salt and pepper and sauté until the veggies are tender, about 5 minutes. Add broth, potatoes, and the lentils. Add Italian seasoning, tomatoes, and spinach. Stir. Bring to a rapid boil over high heat, then cover and simmer over low heat until the lentils are tender, about 40 to 50 minutes.

Ladle in soup bowls, sprinkle with Parmesan cheese and serve.

Veggie (Chicken) Soup

Ingredients:

4 celery stalks, chopped

2 tbsp organic butter

1 medium onion, chopped

6 cloves of garlic, chopped

5 parsley stalks, chopped

1 bag egg noodles (for ketogenic, use zucchini noodles)

salt and pepper to taste

1 tspns Italian Seasoning

1 shredded chicken breast, optional

6-10 cups water bouillon cubes according to package (I try to find one made of all herbs and veggies with the least amount of chemicals.)

1-2 cups carrots, canned or fresh, any style

Directions:

Sauté celery and onions with butter in pot. Add water and bouillon to pot. Bring to boil, adding in noodles. Add all other ingredients. Let simmer for about 15 minutes, or until noodles are done. Let stand until cool enough to eat. Note: This soup can be used as a base for other soups like lentil bean soup or potato soup. Just omit the noodles.

Turkey (or Chicken) Chili

Ingredients:

1 pound ground turkey (or 2 whole chicken breasts)

1 packet organic chili seasoning or 2 tbsp chili powder and ½ tspn cayenne pepper

1 can organic corn

1 can organic black beans (or may substitute 2 cans of Kroger organic tri-beans)

1 can organic red chili beans

1 can organic pinto beans

28 oz canned crushed tomatoes

1 can tomato sauce

Directions:

Brown ground turkey, drain and set aside. In medium pot, add all ingredients. Stir in cooked ground turkey. Let simmer. This can be cooked on stove top or crock pot, on low for 4-6 hours.

I love these recipes that you can literally throw all kinds of good stuff in! I like to sauté some chopped red onion, garlic, and chopped mushrooms in coconut oil, then using the same pan, brown the ground turkey (or whatever meat you're using). Then, when I'm adding all ingredients into the crockpot, I add a little zucchini and/or yellow squash.
MMMmmmmm! (Keep in mind when adding more ingredients, you may need to add in more liquid. I just add in another can of crushed tomatoes or tomato sauce. You can also use a broth.)

Of course, top this bowl off with your favorite
toppings like sour cream, green onions,
crackers, and cheese. I like to also add avocado.

Main Dishes

Sour Kraut and Red Potatoes

Ingredients:

4 medium red potatoes, quartered into bite size pieces

1-2 tablespoons coconut oil or real butter for cooking potatoes

2 tablespoons sweet onion, chopped

3 garlic cloves, minced

1 package Applegate Chicken & Apple Sausage (or any nitrate-free sausage), sliced in bite size pieces

1 jar organic (live) sour kraut

1 medium organic red apple, sliced (optional)

Directions:

In large pan, cook potatoes in coconut oil or butter until almost done. I add a little bit of water to the pan and throw a lid on them. Toss in chopped onions and minced garlic. When potatoes feel almost done, add in sliced Chicken

& Apple sausage. Add in apple slices. Cook until meat is heated through. Finally add in sour kraut. Mix all ingredients together. Add salt and pepper to taste. Enjoy!

Sour kraut is belly good!! Fermented foods are known to have beneficial probiotics that helps to improve digestion, immune function, and so much more! It is perfectly fine to omit the potatoes for a more carb-limited option. It still tastes just as great!

Broccoli Cheese Stuffed Chicken Breast

Ingredients:

2 large chicken breasts

salt & pepper to taste

½ tsp garlic powder

½ tsp Italian seasoning

1 garlic clove, chopped

1 cup finely chopped broccoli florets

2 tbsp finely chopped celery

2 tbsp shaved carrot strings

1 cup mild cheddar cheese

1-2 tbsp mayo

1 tbsp coconut oil

Directions:

Preheat oven to 425 degrees F.

Season both sides of the chicken breasts with salt, pepper, Italian seasoning and ½ tsp of the garlic powder. Use a sharp knife to cut a slice through the middle of the chicken breasts, but not all the way through, creating a pocket for the filling.

For the filling:

In a mixing bowl, add the broccoli, celery, carrot shreds, cheese, mayo, chopped garlic and salt and pepper to taste. Mix until well combined. (This filling made enough for 2-4 chicken breasts, depending on how "stuffed" you want them.)

Heat a skillet over medium heat and add the coconut oil. Sear the chicken for 3 to 4 minutes on each side. Divide the mixture and stuff the two chicken breasts, using a toothpick to secure if necessary. Place stuffed chicken breasts on pie plate cooking stone and bake in preheated oven for about 30 minutes, or until chicken reads 165 degrees. Let rest for 5 minutes before diving in.

Lemon Chicken and Cauliflower Rice

Ingredients

1 tablespoons coconut oil or avocado oil

2 tablespoons real butter

1/2 medium onion, chopped

4 cloves garlic, minced

1/4 teaspoons Italian seasoning

1 bag cauliflower rice, thawed

1 cup filtered water

2 bouillon cubes (I use dried herbs and
seasonings bouillon, not the chemical crap)

1 pound asparagus, cut into bite sized pieces

2 tablespoons lemon juice

1 cup heavy whipping cream

2 cups cooked shredded or rotisserie chicken

1/2 cup Parmesan cheese, grated

Salt and pepper to taste

Directions

Add in oil, butter, and onion to pan over medium heat. Sauté onion for 3-4 minutes.

Add garlic, Italian seasoning, cauliflower rice, water, and bouillon. Stir, then add in asparagus. Cover with lid and cook until asparagus is fork-tender.

Add in the rest of the ingredients except for the chicken. Stir to combine. Then add in the chicken. Cover again until heated through.

Serve with additional lemon slice and Parmesan cheese.

Keto Bread

This recipe yields to one ramekin. I make this recipe one by one ramekin, then bake them all together on a cookie sheet.

Ingredients:

1 large egg

2 tbsp almond flour

1 tbsp real butter

1 tbsp almond milk

¼ tspn baking powder

1/8 tspn real salt

Variations to above recipe:

¼ tspn Italian seasoning, 1/8 tspn garlic powder, can top off with shredded cheddar cheese (optional)

1 tbsp chopped bacon or ham

1 tbsp shredded cheese of your choice

¼ cup finely chopped spinach, 1 tbsp crumbled feta cheese

1 tbsp finely chopped broccoli

Have fun creating your own flavor keto bread!

Instructions:

Preheat the oven to 400 degrees

Grease ramekins with butter or use cooking spray

In a separate (small) mixing bowl, add in all ingredients. Use a fork to or small whisk to completely mix together. This makes one ramekin at a time.

Pour the mixture into a greased ramekin.

Bake for 10-15 minutes

When the bread is done baking, let the ramekins cool. Then, turn over the ramekins to release the bread. Serve with butter at your next meal!

Sweet Treats

Keto "Frosty" Copycat

Ingredients:

<u>Refrigerated</u>

2 cups heavy whipping cream

<u>Condiments</u>

3 tablespoons Swerve Sweetener, granular

<u>Baking & Spices</u>

2 tablespoons organic cocoa powder

2 teaspoons Vanilla extract, pure

Pinch of Redmonds Real Salt

<u>Toppings</u>

Lily's brand Dark Chocolate Chips

Unsweetened Coconut Flakes

Instructions:

Blend in a bowl with a mixer until just before high peaks form. Then, refrigerate. Serve cold and add toppings if desired.

Keto Cheesecake Fluff

Ingredients:

<u>Refrigerated</u>

8 ounces cream cheese, softened

1 cup heavy whipping cream

<u>Condiments</u>

¼ cup Swerve Sweetener, granular

<u>Baking & Spices</u>

1 ½ teaspoons Vanilla extract, pure

<u>Toppings</u>

Lily's brand Dark Chocolate Chips

Unsweetened Coconut Flakes

Instructions:

Beat cream cheese with Swerve, vanilla with an electric mixer until well combined.

In separate bowl, beat heavy cream with mixer until stiff peaks form.

Fold the whipped cream into cream cheese mixture until well incorporated.

Beat with an electric mixer on high until light and fluffy.

Refrigerate for at least two hours. Pipe or spoon into individual serving dishes. Top with sugar-free chocolate, if desired. (If not following keto, you can top with fresh fruit or chocolate sauce and/or peanut butter chips.)

Keto-Layered Fudge

My family has been making the other version of this fudge since I was a little girl. I loved it so much that I had to make a healthier version to keep the tradition going. Give it a try!

Ingredients:

Nut butter fudge

½ cup of your favorite nut butter

½ cup homemade sweetened condensed milk (see recipe on this page)

½ teaspoon vanilla extract

Directions:

Combine the warmed sweetened condensed milk with nut butter and vanilla, stirring until well combined.

Place into silicone mold or 8x8" pan lined with parchment paper. Place in freezer to set.

Chocolate fudge

1 cup Lily's chocolate chips

1 cup homemade sweetened condensed milk (see recipe on this page)

½ teaspoon vanilla extract

Directions:

Melt chocolate chips in pan or double boiler, stirring often to distribute heat. When melted, stir in vanilla, and sweetened condensed milk. Mix until well combined. Take out nut butter fudge and pour the chocolate fudge over it. Set back in freezer to set, about 20 minutes. Then place in refrigerator until ready to serve. Cut into bit size pieces.

Note: Both of these recipes can be made separately or layered together like this to make different desserts.

Nut-Butter Cheesecake Keto Bites

These are a delicious, no-bake, low-carb, high-fat keto dessert that everyone will just love. I made these for our holiday dessert, and everyone just ate them up!

You will need:

8 oz cream cheese, softened

¼ cup Swerve sweetener

1 tsp vanilla extract

¼ cup heavy whipping cream

¼ cup natural peanut butter (or nut butter
of your choice)

¾ cup Lily's Sugar Free chocolate chips

2 tsp coconut oil

Directions:

Mix cream cheese, Swerve, and heavy whipping cream until smooth with a blender. Mix in peanut butter and vanilla extract until fully combined, set aside. Melt chocolate and coconut oil together. Pour into the bottoms only of mini (non-bleached, natural) baking cups.

Place a couple spoonful's of cheesecake fluff into cup and freeze for 15 minutes.

Top cups with chocolate chips or melted chocolate swirls for decoration.

Freeze for 20 minutes covered or refrigerate for 1 hour.

I made about 24 of these from this batch.

Substitutes I Love

Substitutes are a good thing, especially when it comes to sugar. Stevia, for example, is not recognized as sugar in our bodies so it does not raise insulin levels. It makes a great way to swap out regular cane sugar with something sweet. Stevia is much sweeter than regular sugar so keep in mind that a little tiny bit goes a long way.

I know that many people don't like the after-taste that stevia leaves behind. Sometimes I notice it and sometimes I don't. Play around with your recipes to make adjustments. I prepare my own real lemonade in mason jars. I simply add one packet of organic stevia to a one-quart jar. Then, two or three slices of organic lemon. (You can add more slices of lemon if you like a stronger lemon flavor.) Finally, I fill with filtered water. Shake it up to mix. You can drink as is, add ice cubes for immediate chill, or my favorite, let sit in the fridge overnight to allow all three ingredients to really infuse with each other. This makes for a wonderful summertime treat that's also hydrating, cleansing, and refreshing!

Other sugar substitutes I love using are Monk Fruit sweeteners and Swerve sweeteners. These are made from fruits.

Bonus! Fruit Salsa

If your family gatherings are anything like mine, there will never be a shortage of sweet treats and desserts to eat. If you want to add something a bit healthier and just as sweet, try fruit salsa! There are so many ways you can vary this by adding in your family's favorite fruits. Here's how I make mine, complete with cinnamon-sugar chips!

Ingredients:

CINNAMON CHIPS

10 flour tortillas

Room temp grass-fed butter or organic coconut oil

Sugar substitute, like Monk Fruit or Swerve for sugar replacement

Cinnamon for sprinkling

FRUIT SALSA

2 Granny Smith apples, organic

1 lemon

1 cup finely diced melon

1 cup finely diced kiwi

1 lb strawberries

½ lb raspberries

4 tablespoons organic mixed-berry fruit preserves

Directions:

CINNAMON CHIPS

Preheat oven to 350 degrees. Working with two tortillas at a time, lather butter over tortilla shells. Sprinkle sugar substitute over it, then sprinkle cinnamon. Flip each tortilla and repeat. Stack both tortillas on top of each other. Using a pizza cutter, slice through the tortillas, cutting them into bite size (12) wedges. (Like chips.) Place on baking sheet and bake for about 10 minutes, or until crisp.

FRUIT SALSA

Finely chop the apples. Squeeze the juice from one lemon over the apples to prevent browning. Finely chop the rest of the fruit. Combine together in one bowl. Add preserves and mix well. Allow to sit for about 15 minutes before refrigerating to let the ingredients meld together.

I've served this both, as an appetizer and as a dessert. Both went over really well!

Did you know that this book is followed by journals? I have created these journals to aid in the mindfulness for everything from the holistic lifestyle change to weight loss (or weight gain as in my daughter's case), to track calories, sugar, and protein grams and such, but also the mood you're in while eating. They include a daily gratitude section, an "I am" affirmation section, and positive quotes for every day.

There's even a journal to remember those favorite meals; the food that was prepared and the people who shared in the meal, complete with space to add your favorite pic of the meal! I hope you enjoy them as much as my family and I have.

Celebrate everything; find peace, and smile.

Other books titled by Laura B. Hill

Tara's Choice: A Mother-Daughter Cancer Journey

Journal Therapy! Six Week Edition

Journal Therapy to a Healthier You!

Journal to a Healthier You!

The Family Recipe Journal

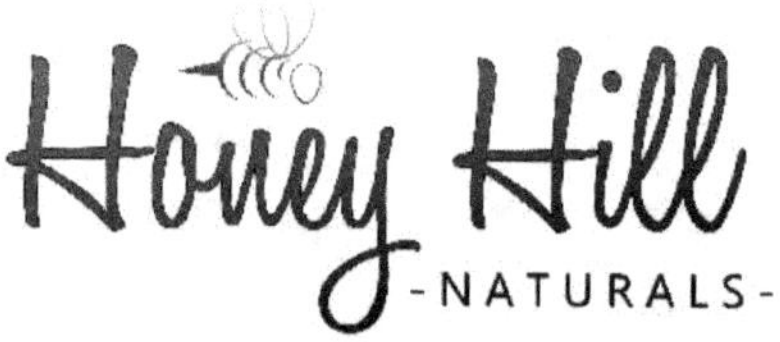

www.onetarahill.org

#onetarahill

Websites Used

"New Study Shows Humans Are on Autopilot Nearly Half the Time."
<https://www.psychologytoday.com/blog/your-brain-work/201011/new-study-shows-humans-are-autopilot-nearly-half-the-time> web. 31 December 2017.

"You Autopilot Mode is Real-Now We Know How the Brain Does it."
<https://www.newscientist.com/article/2151137-your-autopilot-mode-is-real-now-we-know-how-the-brain-does-it/ > 28 October 2017. Web. 31 December 2017.

"How Does Your Stomach Tell Your Brain That You're Full?"
<https://www.livestrong.com/article/489875-how-does-your-stomach-tell-your-brain-that-youre-full/> 18 July 2017. Web. 31 December 2017.

"How to Make Sure You're Eating High-Vibrational Food."
<https://www.mindbodygreen.com/0-11996/how-to-make-sure-youre-eating-

highvibrational-food.html> 17 December 2013. Web. 16 January 2018.

"The Metaphysics of Emotions – Emotional Energy is Real."
<http://joy2meu.com/emotional_energy.htm l> 26 February 2013. Web. 17 January 2018.

"10 Reasons to avoid GMOs"
<http://responsibletechnology.org/10-reasons-to-avoid-gmos/>_25 August 2011. Web. 21 February 2018.

"Cancer is a Preventable Disease that Requires Major Lifestyle Changes." <
https://www.ncbi.nlm.nih.gov/pmc/articles/P MC2515569/> 25 September 2008. Web. 22 March 2018.

"Toxic Chemicals." <
http://wwf.panda.org/about_our_earth/teac her_resources/webfieldtrips/toxics/> Web. 22 March 2018.

"The Inside Story: A Guide to Indoor Air Quality." < https://www.epa.gov/indoor-air-quality-iaq/inside-story-guide-indoor-air-quality> Web. 22 March 2018.

"Why (Most) Sunscreen is Harmful." <https://wellnessmama.com/55366/sunscreen-is-harmful/> 11 January 2018. Web. 28 March 2018.

"Herb Healers, Specials and Bundles." <https://www.herbhealers.com/specials-and-bundles> Web. 28 March 2018.